"Some books stay with you long after the last page; this is one. Having already dedicated their lives and careers to the cause of reproductive freedom, Curtis Boyd and Glenna Halvorson-Boyd have given the world yet another gift with this profoundly moving and beautifully written memoir. *We Choose To* is a story of love, shared humanity, and the power of choosing to stare injustice in the face and do something about it."

—Cecile Richards, former President of Planned Parenthood
and *New York Times* bestselling author of *Make Trouble:*
Standing Up, Speaking Out, and Finding the Courage to Lead

"This intimate and moving account of the reality of abortion care tells a unique story. The authors poetically describe the love and compassion—for their patients, for their staff, and for each other—that drives their work and also grapple with the grim reality for their family of choosing this line of work, as the danger and violence of anti-abortion activists are ever present. Their humility and dedication provide a model that should guide the next generation of abortion providers and advocates."

—Nancy Northup, President and CEO
of the Center for Reproductive Rights

"This memoir from two of the National Abortion Federation's founding members provides a valuable history of abortion provision in freestanding clinics and the pioneering development of abortion counseling amid the backdrop of our country's changing legal landscape. Writing alternating chapters, Curtis and Glenna share the philosophy and rituals they used to establish a patient-centered way of providing abortion care. This book offers an accessible and engaging education about the evolution of in-clinic abortion care in the United States and reads as a love letter to the thousands of patients who taught the authors and their staff so much along the way."

—Melissa Fowler, Chief Program Officer,
National Abortion Federation (NAF)

T0190914

"*We Choose To* is a must-read for anyone curious about the ways that faith impacts abortion care. The memoir reminds readers that religious belief compels many of the physicians, nurses, doulas, counselors, and administrative staff who kept clinics running before, during, and after Roe. The book shows how Dr. Curtis Boyd, a former preacher 'raised on black-eyed peas, corn pone, and Bible verses,' found a new ministry providing abortions. Together, Dr. Boyd and Dr. Halvorson-Boyd share the profoundly moving work of providing lifesaving healthcare in the Deep South."

—Jamie L. Manson, M.Div., President of Catholics for Choice

"*We Choose To* shows us that abortion care is freedom and love, and that abortion providers are compassionate frontline heroes working in a terrain that is increasingly hostile for providers, patients, and their loved ones. What a wonderful reminder that this battle for reproductive freedom and justice did not begin and end with the fall of *Roe v. Wade!*"

—Fatima Goss Graves, President and CEO,
National Women's Law Center

"Curtis Boyd and Glenna Halvorson-Boyd have committed their lives to a shared cause: helping women end the pregnancies they wish to end. But if that commitment made them leaders of the pro-choice movement, this book is no screed. It is an honest look at their difficult work, and it shies away from nothing."

—Joshua Prager, Pulitzer Prize finalist for
The Family Roe: An American Story

"*We Choose To* is the most satisfying love story I've ever read. The Boyds invite the reader into intimate conversation about the spiritual joy of devoting one's life to service, the intellectual passion of creating new medical procedures and counseling approaches, the healthy self-love fueling the choices of both abortion patients and providers, and the way two fiercely independent people can function as soulmates. An essential 'behind the scenes' history of US abortion care from its pioneers, and a manual for how people working for social justice in hard times might sustain themselves and each other."

—Katie Watson, Associate Professor, Feinberg School of Medicine, Northwestern University, and author of *Scarlet A: The Ethics, Law, and Politics of Ordinary Abortion*

"Curtis Boyd and Glenna Halvorson-Boyd have each played hugely significant roles in the evolution of abortion care in the United States. Their contributions include both key medical improvements in abortion methods and new approaches to abortion counseling, as well as to the often-overlooked issue of staff care. In this beautifully written memoir, the reader is introduced to both the challenges and gratifications of a lifetime spent doing this essential work. A bonus feature is the book's moving portrayal of a loving marriage that is able to withstand the stresses of its partners' involvement in the most contentious issue in American politics."

—Carole Joffe, Professor of Obstetrics, Gynecology, and Reproductive Sciences, University of California San Francisco and coauthor of *Obstacle Course: The Everyday Struggle to Get an Abortion in California*

"*We Choose To* tells the story of Glenna and Curtis Boyd, who spent their lives providing much-needed abortion care to women across the country. The book offers a rare look inside a medical practice started by Curtis Boyd in the late 1960s when he was asked to provide underground abortion services as part of the Clergy Consultation Service. And it follows Curtis after abortion becomes legal in 1973 when he meets Glenna, who establishes abortion counseling at his clinics.

As a couple, the two worked on the frontier of providing compassionate abortion care, and the book documents how their moral and religious beliefs guided the services they established. *We Choose To* illustrates what anti-abortion activists try to deny: that abortion care can be tender and restore women's sense of self. It is a rare historical document about an often-hidden medical practice that demonstrates why access to compassionate abortion services is so crucial to women's health and lives."

—Johanna Schoen, Professor of History, Rutgers University
and author of *Abortion After Roe*

"Curtis and Glenna Boyd are heroes of the abortion movement. They have helped many thousands of women with exceptional care. They inspired and taught generations of abortion providers with their unique, courageous, and profoundly empathic practice in the face of unrelenting harassment and political interference."

—Philip Darney, MD and Uta Landy, PhD, Bixby Center for Global Reproductive Health, University of California San Francisco

WE CHOOSE TO

A Memoir of Providing Abortion Care
Before, During, and After Roe

WE CHOOSE TO

Dr. Curtis Boyd, MD, and
Dr. Glenna Halvorson-Boyd, PhD, RN

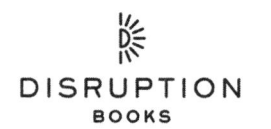

DISRUPTION
BOOKS

New York, NY | Washington, DC

To Pearl "Mama" Boyd,
Mary Funston Halvorson,
and Glenn Halvorson

Published by Disruption Books
Washington, DC
www.disruptionbooks.com

Copyright 2024 by Curtis Boyd and Glenna Halvorson-Boyd

Distributed by Disruption Books
For information about special discounts for bulk purchases, please contact
Disruption Books at info@disruptionbooks.com.

Cover by Emily Mahon and Brian Phillips Design
Author portrait by Jamey Stillings
Book interior design by Jess LaGreca, Mayfly book design

Library of Congress Cataloging-in-Publication Data is available
Printed in the United States of America

Print ISBN: 978-1-63331-087-2
eBook ISBN: 978-1-63331-088-9

First Edition

Contents

December 25, 1988

Glenna

We'd had a perfect Christmas Eve in Santa Fe, New Mexico. Our youngest son, Kyle, was home from university, and after an early dinner we'd bundled ourselves against the cold and walked through the city's historic Eastside neighborhood for hours. The night was clear, the sky was filled with stars, and the streets were lined with tiny handmade lanterns, *farolitos*, their candles burning bright within brown paper bags. Larger fires marked street corners—luminarias of carefully stacked logs where carolers gathered to sing and neighbors shared hot cider or chocolate. Those flames meant warmth; looking back they could be seen as premonition.

When the phone woke me in the middle of the night, I knew it could only be bad news. Still, the words stunned me: "We've had a fire . . ." It was our trusted CEO, Emerson, and my eyes filled with tears.

Christmas Eve and another abortion clinic set ablaze was an old story, even then. But that night, the clinic burning was ours. "Anyone hurt?"

"No."

"Good." Now I could go numb and shift into action mode—my classic defense against horrors. It comes in handy.

Within minutes I was on the phone, booking the first flight back to Dallas. Our Christmas in Santa Fe was over, and the holiday would forever hold a different meaning in our lives.

1

When we arrived in Dallas, we learned there had been three suspicious fires that night—all at Dallas clinics providing abortion care. They fit the pattern of Christmas arson attacks that began in Pensacola, Florida, in 1984, when the arsonists proudly claimed their handiwork as gifts to the baby Jesus. Like many of the Christmas arsons that followed, ours would never be solved.

The police guard on duty at the clinic met us in the back parking lot. In the slanting afternoon light of winter, we walked the perimeter of the building toward what had once been the administrative office at the rear. Portions of the pitched roof had collapsed atop the remains of batten board walls, insulation, and sheetrock. Desks, chairs, typewriters, file cabinets, and huge shards of plate glass that had once been windows poked out of the blackened heap.

"This is where the fire was set," the officer explained. A patch of grass and a wooden fence along the alley had been doused with gasoline, then lit.

I had expected a dismal scene, but somehow the reality was even more wrenching, in part because Kyle was with us. I had always hoped to protect our children—a futile wish but one I'd clung to nonetheless. Providing abortions had been our career choice, not theirs. Kyle's older brother and sister were far away, launching their own interesting careers. Kyle was spending Christmas Day at a crime scene, and I was heartsick.

Curtis

We followed the police officer deeper into the ruins. The clinic had been a two-story, wood-frame house that I repurposed in 1973 as the first legal abortion facility in the US Southwest. The administrative office was an addition, separated from the medical offices by a solid wall of concrete blocks, which had served as a firewall. Without it, the entire building would have been consumed.

We entered the clinic through what had been the back door, now broken down by firefighters. The officer gave us flashlights, and their beams guided us through an eerie landscape of familiar rooms and furniture. Water was puddled on the linoleum floor of the surgery and lab rooms. As we picked our way into the recovery room, with its carpeted floor and comfortable wraparound sofa intended to signal to patients that they were back to everyday life, the carpeting squished underfoot.

Walking along the hallway to the waiting room, furnished like a living room in an inviting home, we saw that patches of wall were smudged with soot that had been carried from the back office through the shared ventilation system. Up the spiral stairs to the second floor's more private counseling areas, the scene was even worse. In addition to the water damage and grayed walls, an indefinable stench—burned plastics, wood, and composite shingles—permeated the place: the smell of destruction.

We were relieved that the Dallas Fire Department had saved the clinic and that no one was hurt. We always closed at that time of year so staff could have truly happy holidays and we could have family time. Still, we were shaken.

Kyle, who had long known about and supported our work, felt worried for us in ways he'd never expressed. I had performed my first abortion in the year Kyle was born. Now, as we stood in the parking lot at dusk, breathing fresh air in gulps, he said, "Do you have to keep doing this work?"

Glenna and I were silent for a long moment. Then I simply said, "No. We choose to."

Part I

Our Lives

CHAPTER ONE

A Girl Named Sallie: Finding Myself, Finding My Calling

"The cycle of life is a puzzling thing; birth, life, death. . . .
I look back on my choice and the path I have made, and think
of the great distance I have traveled. This I will never forget."
—*Patient journal entry*

Curtis

Her name was not Sallie, but whenever my father couldn't remember a girl's name, that's what he'd call her. I forgot this Sallie's name on purpose, for her privacy and my own protection, but I'll never forget her.

As soon as my nurse showed her into the consultation room, I knew she was a poor farm girl, seventeen years old at most. With stringy hair and no makeup, a feed sack dress, and shoes cobbled from worn-out boot soles tied on with homemade strips of leather, she could have stepped out of a Faulkner novel. By contrast, I was the picture of small-town success: clean-shaven face, military-short haircut, black horn-rimmed glasses, and a white shirt with a tie knotted firmly at the collar.

It was 1967, and I was a thirty-year-old doctor with a thriving private practice in the small town of Athens, Texas, seventy miles east of Dallas.

She was not one of my patients, but we had more in common than our appearances would suggest. We came from the same part of the world—rural East Texas, where we'd both been raised on black-eyed peas, corn pone, and Bible verses. Like her, I had grown up in the countryside, seven miles outside Athens by a farm-to-market road, then three miles down a dirt track. I imagined that Athens, population five thousand at the time, seemed like a metropolis to Sallie, as it had seemed to me when I was young. That she had come to town by herself was reason to take notice.

I invited her to take a seat. "What can I do for you, Sallie?"

She wasted no time with niceties. "I need you to do me an abortion."

In 1967, abortion was a felony offense in forty-nine states plus the District of Columbia. Later that year, Colorado would be the first state to decriminalize the procedure, but we were in Texas, where people followed the *Farmers' Almanac* more closely than the national news and listened to Christian hymns more than Beatles tunes. And because many of my patients knew I had been a preacher before I became a physician, they trusted me to provide a bit of wisdom from both professions. When medicine failed to restore an aging matriarch or revive a stillborn, my patients asked me to pray with them and then said, "Thank you, brother." We were all brothers and sisters in Christ, and to many, I was as much brother as doctor.

Personally and politically, I supported the idea of abortion rights—even discussed the possible benefits of legalization with classmates in medical school—but I'd never performed an abortion, and I had never considered doing one in my family practice. I was a responsible, respected member of the community with a good livelihood and a bright future. I had a wife and three young children to support. This girl had no idea what she was asking of me.

My answer was simple: "I can't. It's illegal."

Sallie was unmoved. "I don't care, 'cause I gotta have one."

I should have asked her to leave, but something stopped me. Perhaps it was her determination. She was a force, to be sure. But there was something more, something that came from inside me—a memory.

As a sophomore, I had transferred to Athens High School after my small country school had burned down. I went from a class of twelve students, all of whom I'd known since first grade, to a class of one hundred students, all strangers. I was still learning the social ropes of the "big city" school when I met Barbara in algebra class. She was pretty, smart, and a little shy, and I helped her with homework several times after school. I remember telling a new friend that I wanted to take her on a date.

He laughed. "You can't date her," he said. "She got knocked up. She has a kid at home."

I hadn't known. No wonder she was shy and all too grateful for my help. She was an outcast. Meanwhile, the boy who everyone knew had impregnated her might as well have won a trophy. In fact, he did win a trophy—in football—and an appointment to West Point when he graduated.

Barbara was just one of several girls I knew who got pregnant in high school. These girls disappeared for a time, and when they returned, they either had a baby or they did not. There was a rumor that a doctor in a nearby town provided illegal abortions, but for a hefty price: $500. (That is the equivalent of between $4,000 and $5,000 in the early 2020s.) Such sums were out of reach for most people of my community. In my youth, women didn't get abortions even if someone was willing to provide one, because they couldn't afford it. Abortion was not yet a political or religious cause, but because it was illegal, it was cloaked in secrecy and myth. What we did know was that women who had sex before marriage and got pregnant were to be shunned. They were soiled goods.

I liked Barbara, but when my friend told me that she had a baby, I did what was expected. I did not ask her out, and my crush faded. Still, I knew it wasn't right or fair that she should be treated like an outcast, and I felt that something should be done to right this wrong. At the time, though, I had no idea what that would be.

I had no further contact with Barbara during high school. Then, in 1967—a few months before Sallie came to my office—I met Barbara again. Her parents were patients of mine, and she came to my office after her father had a heart attack. Despite the unhappy circumstances, I looked forward to seeing her again. I imagined that I would tell her what I could not say in high school: that I'd had a crush on her, that I knew she'd been mistreated. But the woman who came to my office bore little resemblance to the high school girl I fondly remembered. This woman was angry; she wore the deep lines of a permanent scowl. When I realized she didn't even remember me, I shifted to professional mode. But seeing her like that stuck with me.

Sallie brought back the ache of that memory. I couldn't help but wonder if Barbara's bitterness was a result of having been treated like a pariah in high school. I could do nothing for her back then, but would I help Sallie now?

"Well, let me examine you first to see if you're pregnant," I said.

"I know I am," she insisted, climbing onto the exam table. "I already told you. I know when it happened—eight weeks ago."

Sallie did not tell me the circumstances surrounding her pregnancy or how she knew the exact day of conception, and I didn't ask. But I could see she was desperate. She was alone and penniless. No one in her family knew she was in Athens seeking help. If I helped her, I would risk my reputation in this small town, my medical license, and thus the welfare of my family, not to mention my freedom.

As I carefully performed a pelvic exam to confirm what she already knew, verses from an old hymn played in my mind:

Hungry and faint and poor,
Behold us, Lord, again
Assembled at Thy mercy's door,
Thy bounty to obtain.

Thy word invites us nigh
Or we must starve indeed;

For we no money have to buy,
No righteousness to plead.

This girl needed help, and I could help her. I knew what I would do before I could admit it to myself.

. . . .

How long was Sallie in my office? I can't recall, but it wasn't long. When I look back now, I marvel at the speed with which I made a plan.

In the 1960s, D&C (dilation and curettage) procedures were performed in a hospital operating room with full anesthesia for women who were diagnosed with an incomplete miscarriage or unexplained bleeding. I could get Sallie admitted to the hospital for a D&C without stirring up suspicion. As a family doctor in a small town, I was on call in the emergency room several days each month, including the following day. Thanks to my reputation, no one would question my medical judgment.

In minutes, I'd worked out the puzzle. "We have never met. You do not know me, understand?" I said.

"Yes," Sallie replied.

"Go to the hospital at 8:00 a.m. tomorrow and tell the emergency room nurse you are bleeding and cramping with a miscarriage. When she asks who your doctor is, tell her you don't have one. I am the doctor on call, so she will call me, and I will come to admit you."

Sallie agreed to the plan and left my office. I didn't know where she went, and I didn't ask. The less I knew, the better.

The next morning, as expected, the nurse called. "Dr. Boyd, Sallie Fuller is in the emergency room, and she says that you're going to admit her for an abortion."

This was definitely not the plan.

"Sallie who?" I asked. "I don't know anything about this."

The nurse asked what she should do.

I took a deep breath and said, "Send her to my office."

When Sallie arrived, I made sure the door to the consultation room was closed. I was angry. But Sallie was angrier—why hadn't I met her at the hospital?

"Because you didn't stick to the plan," I explained. "No one must know I'm doing an abortion. Now we have a problem."

She remained determined. "You gonna do it for me."

I admitted her to the hospital with a diagnosis of "inevitable miscarriage." I had no trouble arranging for a surgery room and anesthesia. With a nurse assisting me, performing the abortion was surprisingly easy, but I knew I couldn't pull that off more than once.

Sallie stayed overnight at the hospital as D&Cs were considered serious surgeries at the time. I instructed her to return to my office for a follow-up; I wanted to help her with birth control. But she didn't come. I neither saw nor heard from her again. Sallie remained a stranger—all but an apparition. I had no idea that, like Barbara, she would haunt me in the years to come.

. . . .

I grew up on my father's and grandfather's farm. In my world, only men were landowners. Like other children in that rural community, I worked long hours caring for livestock and tilling the land. I studied hard in school and went to church regularly—the third weekend of each month, when the circuit preachers came to the one-room church on my grandfather's land. My family belonged to the Primitive Baptist Church of Predestinarian Faith and Order, also known as the "foot-washing Baptists," a small fundamentalist sect that believes—above all else—that our lives are predetermined by God.

I studied the Bible as a child. If I had a talent, it was for remembering what I read. I could recite chapter and verse with ease and did so during church services. I might have been showing off, but my grandmother believed my behavior was evidence that I had been called by God to some special purpose. "Mama Boyd" was my anchor. She could both cure warts with knots in a dishrag by the light of the moon and hold a faith in me as absolute as her faith in God.

By the time I was in high school, the elders of the church decided I had been "called" to preach. I traveled with my father to other small churches in the region to extemporaneously speak the Word of God and defend the faith. In my community, to be chosen to preach was the highest calling, and I did my best to live up to expectations, but I had doubts even then.

The values taught in my faith didn't always align with the values I saw lived out in my community. If all were equal in God's eyes, why were some of His children required to drink from a different water fountain or use a different bathroom? Although I wanted to remain among the faithful—they were my people, and the church was a central part of our culture—on the inside I was filled with doubts. I raised such questions only in silent conversations with myself, however, as I walked the woods and fields.

My father, who had served as a training officer in the military, understood the value of a higher education and had saved money to send me to university. I was the first person in my family to get such an education. Once away at Texas A&M, I was exposed to new ways of thinking. In the library I was shocked to learn that the Bible had not been originally written in King James's English. I had a physics professor who publicly declared that he was an atheist—the first atheist I had ever met—and I thought him a decent human being. It was liberating but also disturbing. As my commitment to critical, scientific thinking deepened, it became more painful to preach in the small rural churches when I'd return home.

I could no longer blindly embrace the faith, but I still felt bound by the rules of my culture. Thus, during my senior year at A&M, I married LaMerle, a girl (that was the word used at the time) I had met on a blind date on one of my visits home. In our world, early marriage was expected. Girls grew up to be wives and mothers; boys became husbands and fathers—and the sole provider for the family, if they were to maintain that family's honor. These were expectations to be met, roles to be fulfilled, and that's as far as I thought about the matter. I accepted my new responsibility to LaMerle, but my priority continued to be my education for my future career in medicine.

When I graduated from medical school in 1963, I hoped to do a residency in internal medicine and pursue a career in academic medicine, but my father didn't have the money for further training. So, after graduation, I returned to my hometown to open a family practice with my friend Ben Johnson. We had met in the Corp of Cadets at Texas A&M and became as close as brothers during medical school. We did nearly everything together—from selling Bibles door-to-door during summer vacation to studying for our boards after medical school. We both graduated at the top of our medical school class yet were returning to our small-town roots, so it seemed a natural partnership at the time.

Returning to Athens also allowed me to fulfill a fantasy straight out of my favorite *Peanuts* comic strip, published in 1959 during my first semester of medical school. In the cartoon, Linus dreamed that he would become a "world-famous humble little country doctor." Although I was hardly world-famous, I was at the top of my world—a successful doctor, married with children, and a pillar of the Athens community—all before I was thirty years old.

My adult motivations were more complex: I had come home to serve the people who had raised me. But this also meant I had to be the person they expected me to be, and I had sorely misjudged how much I had changed. Although Ben and I were a good team, over time it became apparent that our personal beliefs and values were at odds. Ben remained a fundamentalist Christian and—as I would later discover—was morally opposed to abortion, while I questioned the morality of denying abortion to women in need. Typical of men of our culture and time, Ben and I didn't talk about our differences. We stayed busy serving our patients and our community.

Outside the small world of Athens, the larger world was changing in dramatic ways. The Civil Rights Movement was on the rise, and 1967 (the year I met Sallie) had been a particularly volatile year. During what journalists were calling the "long, hot summer of 1967," some 159 race riots erupted across the nation. For me, those riots happened only on TV, on the evening news from Buffalo or Cincinnati—not in Athens. Dr. Martin Luther King Jr. spoke in Mississippi, Alabama, New York—but not rural Texas.

The feminist movement was taking hold as well. Betty Friedan's *The Feminine Mystique*, published in 1963, was credited with launching the second wave of feminism, which focused on addressing social inequities. (The first wave, which launched at the turn of the twentieth century, tackled legal issues, most famous among them the right to vote.) While it would be years before Athens would feel the ripples from that second wave, I was aware of the call for equality among the sexes. I had managed to get the Pill for LaMerle after the birth of our first son, Curtis Jr., in my final year of medical school. Now I was quietly prescribing it for married women who asked for it, but such requests were not yet common in Athens. The sexual revolution had not reached our town.

In time, I would teach classes in sex education and contraception. Eventually, I would call myself a feminist. But in 1967, when I met Sallie, I still appeared as buttoned-up as my starched white shirt.

I was the county health officer, the owner of a nursing home, and a member of the school board, while LaMerle dutifully fulfilled the role of mother and doctor's wife. We were products of the same rural Texas environment; we understood its rules and could go through the motions. But my increasing commitment to the social activism of the 1960s was changing me. I felt lonely in our marriage, cast in the traditional role of provider with LaMerle and disciplinarian with our children, dissatisfied in ways I couldn't or wouldn't name. I did not talk with LaMerle about my feelings—emotional reflection was never part of our relationship. Instead, I worked long days, racing from the office to the hospital to the nursing home. I remained on call 24/7.

When I could, I'd take an afternoon off, go back to my father's farm to drive the old tractor and mow an acre or two, relieved to be lost in the tasks of childhood. I needed time alone to ponder. How could I have a satisfying life without doing harm to my family?

. . . .

I spoke to no one about Sallie's abortion, but I ruminated on it—both the larger social issue that had troubled me since high school and the logistics. I didn't plan to do another, but merely as a thought experiment, I pondered: How could a family-practice doctor provide safe abortions outside of a hospital? Why had I treated hundreds of abortion complications during my training? Was the procedure really so fraught with medical risks? Equally important, how could a responsible doctor not get caught?

I wondered why a D&C had to be performed in a hospital setting with full anesthesia. The procedure was simple and short. Few instruments were needed, and I could imagine keeping them in my office. I had an autoclave to sterilize instruments, of course. I saw no reason to keep the patient overnight. Yes, pain management could be a problem. Yet I knew some pain could be managed with local anesthesia because I'd done it with obstetric patients. Dentists managed pain in their offices every day.

What of the staff involvement? I could work in the procedure room of my office, with only the patient present. Without an assistant, the procedure would take more time, but it would not be proper to involve my staff in illegal work. They would suspect, of course, just as the staff at the hospital probably did, but a doctor's authority was nearly absolute in those days. The staff would not question me.

Although I thought about all of this, I had no conscious plan to follow through. Instead, I hoped to join forces with like-minded people of faith to change public opinion and the laws. Looking back, I have to laugh at myself.

In university, I'd begun to develop my own brand of faith—my personal religion. The religious beliefs I'd been exposed to while growing up were rooted in dogma and no longer fit my need for a rational belief system. I was seeking truth with a small *t*, not the biblical Truth of my upbringing, and I wanted a faith based on compassion and service to those in need. Then, in medical school, I was introduced to the First

Unitarian Church of Dallas. I was shocked: they had "stolen" my religion! But finally, I could feel at home in a church. It was a welcome contrast to the church of my childhood, to which I would never return. My family, especially Mama Boyd, would forever believe that by becoming a doctor instead of a preacher, I had chosen the lesser calling. I would have to live with the painful knowledge that my beloved grandmother died praying I would see the error of my ways and come home "preaching Jesus Christ and Him crucified."

When I returned to Athens, I joined the Unitarian Fellowship in Tyler, Texas, thirty-five miles east of Athens, and later became its president. Through that fellowship, I met a group of chaplains who were forming a Clergy Consultation Service on Problem Pregnancy (CCS) in Dallas in 1967.[1] The CCS was founded that year in New York City with leadership from the Reverend Howard Moody—who was the senior minister at Judson Memorial Church in Lower Manhattan but had been born a Southern Baptist in Dallas—and the organization quickly grew into a loose network of roughly 1,400 ministers and rabbis all across the United States. These clergy members were working to change laws against abortion and, in the meantime, to refer women to reputable doctors who could help them.

The CCS had a system: A woman seeking an abortion would contact a CCS member—often the chaplain at a local college or university. A volunteer minister or rabbi would meet with the woman to provide counseling, spiritual support, a bus ticket if needed, and the name and address of a licensed doctor. The CCS group in Dallas was looking for doctors to do abortions in the Southwest, and in late 1967 the Reverend Bill Nichols from the Richardson Unitarian Church asked me to aid in their search. Without revealing my encounter with Sallie earlier that same year, I assured him that I was happy to be of service.

While visiting doctors in Texas, I quickly learned that the good ones, if they agreed to speak to me at all, didn't want to take such a risk. Those I met in Mexico were not in fact licensed medical doctors. I was disappointed and disillusioned. Then, in early 1968, the Reverend Robert Cooper, assistant chaplain at Southern Methodist University (SMU), asked if he could come to Athens to talk with me. Although I could guess why he wanted to meet in person, I didn't want to think about it.

Indeed, when he arrived, Reverend Cooper got straight to the point. "We've had no success finding doctors, and we are inundated with requests from desperate women," he said. "Would you consider doing the abortions yourself?"

I thought about Sallie. Once again, I knew that I should say no. I had too many people depending on me, too much at stake. Even if I was willing to take the risk, did the welfare of my family, my three beloved children, take precedence? Caught in a moral dilemma, I asked Reverend Cooper for some time to think about it. But I knew, even before he left my office, that I would risk it all.

· · · ·

As soon as I said yes to Reverend Cooper, pregnant women started coming to our office—one or two women a day at first. It was easy enough to fit these patients into my regular schedule, and no one was the wiser. Before long, however, I was seeing twenty, sometimes thirty women a day. Clearly, there was a great need for abortion care.

My partner, Ben, was busy with his patients; I was busy with mine. I performed the procedures in my examination room, behind closed doors. I could not provide general anesthesia, but I was perfecting my local anesthetic technique. Even when my patients felt pain, they were stoic. After the surgery, which took less than fifteen minutes to perform, the women rested briefly. They were in and out in the time of an average office call. I charged $100 and waived the fee when the patient couldn't afford to pay.

Unlike the shady back-alley affairs that were legend in big cities at the time—where a woman might be blindfolded and taken to an undisclosed location for an abortion performed by an anonymous person whose credentials she could not verify—the women who found me through the CCS knew my name, address, and phone number. Further, they knew that they had ongoing support from the CCS ministers who referred them. This was the furthest thing from the infamous coat-hanger abortion. Yet it was still illegal.

No one on my staff knew I was performing abortions—or if they knew, they didn't say. If Ben noticed how many of my patients were from out of town, he said nothing either. *Don't ask, don't tell* was a rule in our world long before it became US military policy. But it isn't easy keeping a secret in a small town. People notice when you change your shoes, let alone your working habits. Neighbors began to remark on unfamiliar cars with license plates from Dallas or Austin. Rumors spread—mostly specula-tion—and people wondered what I was doing to draw so many strangers to our town. The local police suspected I was dealing drugs. What else would bring young people with out-of-county license tags to my office?

I was careful not to let Ben know what I was doing—in part to protect him and in part to keep our practice alive. I respected him as a colleague and, despite our differences, still loved him like a brother. Living next door to each other in federally subsidized housing throughout medical school had allowed us a rare intimacy. By simply opening our medicine cabinets, we had a window into each other's bathroom. We used these portholes to communicate day and night—whether debriefing a difficult medical case or just to say, "Meet you at the car in ten minutes."

Now we were merely courteous to each other. I was changing. I wore a black armband to show my opposition to the war in Vietnam, and I took Black families to lunch and took their children to the local swim-ming pool to show my support for integration. Neither were popular causes in Athens, but I was no longer courting popularity. I had aban-doned my compliant facade and was openly defying the long-held val-ues of our community—which Ben still upheld, even embodied. I was a liability to our medical practice. Presumably for these reasons, and perhaps more, late in 1968 I returned from a weekend off duty to find a sealed envelope on my desk. The letter was three brief lines:

> *Dear Curtis,*
> *I must end our partnership per the terms of our legal agreement.*
> *Sincerely, Ben*

Ben and I never talked of abortion or the other issues that tore us apart, nor did we speak of the pain our professional split caused us both. Everything remained unspoken, but I read between the lines. For me, it was a divorce. I knew parting ways was for the best: it would protect Ben from any guilt by association if I were caught. And with more and more women coming to my office from all over the region, the likelihood that I'd be discovered increased every day.

By then, I knew that I would not stop seeing abortion patients. I was consumed by the work, moved by the women's stories—and overwhelmed by the number of women who so desperately needed a safe abortion. I could have worked twenty-four hours a day, seven days a week, and still not met the demand. The more patients I saw who needed to terminate their pregnancies, the more I realized that women like Barbara and Sallie were not anomalies. Ill-timed or unhealthy pregnancies affect women of all socioeconomic backgrounds, and of every race and culture, and restrictions on their reproductive rights have far-reaching consequences. Seeing women through this underground network broadened my understanding of what it meant to be a woman in the 1960s and strengthened my belief that I was doing the right thing.

However, I was not ready to leave the only place I'd ever called home. I still wanted to have it both ways: I thought I could remain a respected pillar of the community while blazing a trail for social change. At the end of 1968, I bought Ben out of the practice, "per the terms of our legal agreement," forcing him to set up anew. Although I have long regretted the unnecessary hardship I caused him, Ben built a successful practice. He stayed in Athens for the rest of his life, serving not only our mutual patients but also my family members.

I, on the other hand, would be gone in a year.

. . . .

Late in 1969, a couple arrived in Athens driving a Volkswagen camper van. In those days, only hippies drove VW vans, and there were no hippies in Athens. Perhaps it should have been no surprise then that a

Henderson County sheriff's officer pulled the couple over, searched the vehicle and the driver, and found marijuana.

The man was arrested and taken to jail. The officer did not search the woman, who was allowed to drive the minivan away. Still deemed worthy of suspicion, she sped to my clinic for her scheduled abortion appointment with a police car on her tail. Bursting through the doors, she found me in the hallway.

"Help me get rid of this shit!" the young woman said. She had stuffed bags of marijuana into her purse and shirt, and she needed to get rid of them fast. When I indicated the bathroom down the hall, she pulled me in to help her. As she unloaded her stash, bits of marijuana went everywhere: down her shirt, all over the floor. She took off her blouse and shook it out, sending up clouds of leaves and green dust.

I had little experience with any illicit drugs. Together we attempted to flush her marijuana down the toilet but discovered—to my horror—marijuana floats.

I had patients waiting, so I called in a few of my staff to clean up the mess. It took them thirty minutes, and it took us all deep into illegal territory. Now I had involved my staff in breaking the law, something I had sworn I would never do. And the police car was still out front.

My imagination ran wild: *What if the officer comes inside even without a warrant? What if he calls for backup, and they dig up the septic line and find the marijuana that went down the toilet?* I needed to calm my raging mind. My afternoon schedule was filled with patients, so I did what I have always done: I took a deep breath and got on with the day's work. I performed the young woman's abortion while the police car idled in the parking lot.

Eventually, the police officer left. Shortly after, so did the young woman, and I was never so relieved to see a patient go. But she wasn't gone long. An hour later she returned, this time with a threat from her boyfriend: if I didn't bail him out, he would report me to the police for doing abortions.

The boyfriend reasoned that it was my fault he was in jail. If I hadn't provided abortions, he and his girlfriend would never have come to

Athens. If they hadn't come to Athens, he would not have been arrested. His logic may have been thin, but he knew that I had more to lose than he did. To get them out of my life, I had to get him out of jail.

When I went with the young woman to the jail, the first person I saw was the district attorney, Mack Wallace—a friend and the son of a nurse who had worked for me until her retirement. I felt a flash of panic: Did he know I was coming? Was he waiting for me?

"Curtis, what are you doing here?" the district attorney asked.

A rumor had been going around town about an officer planting drugs on people during routine stops to boost his arrest record. So I told Mack that I was helping a patient whose boyfriend had been arrested for marijuana possession and that I believed the officer had planted the drugs.

"Do you have any proof?" Mack demanded.

"Well, no, only what she tells me."

"You'd better not say that again if you can't prove it," he replied.

This was not our usual friendly banter. The DA's words sounded a warning. His tone said even more: it signaled a change in our relationship and in my standing in the community.

I let the issue drop and paid the boyfriend's bail, and the couple left town. Then I returned to the office, shaken by my exchange with the DA. Suddenly I realized that he would not protect me. For the first time, the risk I was taking felt real and immediate—if caught, I would go to prison.

Preoccupied with my own fears, I hadn't appreciated how distressed my staff was until my senior nurse asked to speak privately the next day. "Dr. Boyd, I believe in what you're doing," she said, without using the A-word, "but you can't keep doing it here. It's time for you to move to the city."

She was right. Looking back, I can't believe I had to wait for someone else to tell me that providing illegal abortions in a small, conservative town in rural East Texas was not sustainable.

As soon as I could, I went to Dallas to look for a new office. Within a day, I found the right spot.

Within a week, with the help of Reggie—a new nurse I'd met through the Unitarian Universalists—I packed a moving van, abandoning the building where Ben and I had started our practice, and moved to the city. Within a day of the move, I started seeing patients.

I took pride in the speed and efficiency with which I made the professional change. But I had put aside any thoughts about the cost to my family. The move to Dallas meant pulling my older children from a cozy small-town school, where they knew all of their classmates and teachers, and thrusting them into the Dallas school system, where everything and everyone was unfamiliar. LaMerle had to leave family and friends she had known all her life, pack up our house, and move to a city where she did not want to live. Although LaMerle supported women's rights, she did not support my choice to break the law. She resented the risk I was taking—with good reason—and worried, even more than I did, about the consequences to our family if I were arrested and jailed.

I was not going to abandon the cause, however, and we saw no better choice for the family. So when I left, LaMerle and the children followed. It seems ironic now that I saw no conflict between my increasingly radical commitment to feminist issues and the assumption that my own traditional male role as head of household and sole decision-maker would continue unchanged. In the feminist ethos of the 1960s, "the personal was political," and change, like charity, began at home. But that ideal was seldom realized—and certainly not in my case. As products of our place and time, both LaMerle and I remained true to our traditional marriage roles. Keeping the family together was a value we still shared even if we resented each other every step of the way.

I reasoned that, in the long run, we would all be safer and thus happier in the big city. I was wrong. In Dallas, I was a stranger with no trusted colleagues and no reputation to fall back on. I was certainly no one's "brother." While I enjoyed relative anonymity, I was no safer there. Although the police were oblivious to my work, to others, I seemed like an easy mark.

One day when I returned from lunch, Reggie said there was a man waiting to talk with me. I asked her to seat him in my office and entered from my private door.

I had no idea who this man was, so I asked, "What can I do for you?"

He pulled a large pistol from under his overcoat and, with a shaking hand, pointed it at my face. "I'm here to rob you," he said.

Oh, damn! was my first thought, but I felt oddly calm. "You must be desperate to do this," I said. "What's wrong?"

"I have five young children," he replied—and I heard the plea. "I can't feed them, and we're about to be evicted. I know you have money because I was here last week with my wife."

Suddenly I understood. A few days earlier, Reggie had mentioned a man with five children sitting in the waiting room while I did his wife's abortion—for free. He had no money then, and he was clearly agitated now.

Just then, the phone rang. "May I answer?" I asked.

He nodded.

It was a friend from a group I'd been out sailing with the past weekend. I'd hurt my back on the boat, and she was calling to see how I was doing.

"Not well," I told her. "I should be home, but I have a full appointment book for two weeks out. All of them are desperate for an abortion. If I don't see these women now, they'll have no chance of a future appointment in time. I can't bear the pain that will cause—for them or me. In fact, I've got to get back to work now."

It was all true, but I was just buying time, hoping the distressed husband would calm down. His agitation made him unpredictable. I was willing to give him money, but I didn't want to get shot.

When I hung up the phone, he said, "I can't do this. May I put the gun away?"

"Yes," I replied. "Please do."

"I'll leave quietly. I won't disturb anyone in your waiting room. OK?"

"I'm sure you won't." I rose and took two hundred-dollar bills from my pocket. "Here, take this."

"No!" he protested. "I can't take your money."

I walked around my desk and shoved the money in his right front pocket, embraced him, and said, "Go in peace, brother. I hope you find help for your family." He quietly left, and I went to the surgery area to begin my afternoon schedule of abortions.

I felt oddly peaceful. A devoted father had done what he thought he needed to do, and I was doing what I needed to do. Maintaining a facade of calm had become second nature, allowing me to wall off my fear. Every day, with every abortion, I faced the possibility that the next patient could send me to prison. That big pistol was just one more threat.

During my time in Dallas, five or six people tried to blackmail me, threatening to report me to the police. It was always the men, the partners of my patients—never the women themselves. Each time, I would insist that as a doctor, I was permitted to speak only with the patient. She was the lone witness, so she would have to file the charge. After repeated menacing phone calls, each man ultimately gave up, but only after I'd say, exasperated, "Go ahead and report me. I see the wives of police officers all the time." That was true but also a bluff—which, fortunately, went in my favor.

I did experience breaks in my calm facade. At times, I imagined that a police car in my rearview mirror was surely tailing me. Occasionally, as I drove to or from work, alone in the eerie light of dawn or dusk, I wondered if I was crazy to persist in this work in the face of constant risk. Then I'd hear another patient's desperate story, see her relief and gratitude when I'd completed her abortion, and lose myself in the task at hand and the larger meaning of the work. Just as each woman had to trust me—a stranger to her—with her life and health, I had to trust the women and families I served. I could not begin to fear them.

At the end of my workday, when everyone was gone and I was alone in the darkened office, I meditated, repeating mantras until I felt able to drive home to my own family. Between all the time I spent working, plus the extra time trying to soothe my own ragged nerves, I often missed dinner with my children, and I was never able to attend their school functions. I did, though, make sure I was home in time to tuck them into bed and tell them bedtime stories. We ended every evening with the same words: "Love and peace. Sweet dreams."

These brief and tender moments aside, my whole family was miserable.

. . . .

Trying to keep a secret in a big city isn't much easier than keeping one in a small town. My name was whispered in certain political and legal circles because wives and girlfriends of policemen and politicians and judges did come to my office for care—which provided a small measure of security. Further, the ministers with the Clergy Consultation Service continued to screen all potential patients, stressing the importance of keeping my name and address confidential. As in Athens, however, I was constantly aware that anyone who came to my office, or even just talked to someone who had, could expose me.

One woman almost did, by trying to use my vulnerability to her advantage. The patient—a woman from Fort Worth who needed an abortion—wasn't the problem. Under normal circumstances, I'd have been happy to help her. But she came with a friend, a woman who was quick to inform me that she was a nurse at John Peter Smith Hospital, where I'd done my postgraduate training. The nurse wanted me to know that she was in charge and ready for any emergency. In fact, in the back of her station wagon, she had installed a bed, an IV pole hung with intravenous fluids, and pain medication—a makeshift ambulance for the ride home.

None of this was necessary for a routine first-trimester abortion. This degree of over-preparedness was curious. It certainly called more attention to the nurse than to the patient. What worried me further was that the nurse had asked her colleagues at John Peter Smith about me and received, in her words, "great reviews." The last straw came when she explained that the Tarrant County district attorney was a mutual friend of ours and that she'd asked for his opinion and received another glowing recommendation.

It seemed as if she had talked to half of Texas about me and my business! I felt confident that she did not report these "reviews" to flatter me. She wanted me to know that she had the upper hand. If the Tarrant

County DA knew I was providing abortions, it might not be long before word spread to Dallas County and District Attorney Henry Wade.

A few years back, Wade had attracted national attention for his prosecution of Jack Ruby for the dramatic jailhouse murder of Lee Harvey Oswald, the accused assassin of President John F. Kennedy. Now Wade was fighting to keep abortion illegal in Texas. He had just filed a case that was on its way to the US Supreme Court in which he was the named defendant: the now-famous *Roe v. Wade*.

The political debate regarding abortion was heating up, and the last place I wanted to be was in the center of the fire. So, for the first time ever, I decided to refuse a patient for a reason that was not medical. I told the woman from Fort Worth that I could not provide the abortion because her friend had involved a host of people, which made it too dangerous for both of us.

"You can't do this!" the friend said, furious. "I'll report you to the district attorney."

It was almost laughable. Did she think I would rather be reported for doing an abortion or for refusing to do one? "I do not know where you received your information, but let me state it clearly," I replied. "I do not perform abortions." I showed the women to the door.

If only that had been the end of it.

The nurse complained about me to several feminist groups in Dallas. She contacted the CCS to report me, and I doubted that she was finished. She had involved so many people that I believed I could no longer stay in Dallas. I needed to get out of the big city and go someplace quieter, safer.

Within a day of the women's visit to my office, I decided to move.

New Mexico had decriminalized "medically justified" abortion the previous year. This law was complicated in practice, but it provided a ray of hope and a path out of Dallas and its inherent dangers. So, by the end of 1970—barely a year after we arrived in the city—I uprooted my family once again. This time we moved to Santa Fe.

Snow lay on the ground the day we arrived—more snow than I had ever seen in my life. The high desert landscape, the low adobe architecture, and the tolerant attitudes of the people were unlike anything I'd known in Texas. I set up a clinic in an old adobe house not far from the Plaza, the heart of downtown Santa Fe. For the first time in years, I didn't worry about the police raiding my clinic. I didn't worry about extortion or blackmail. I relaxed, let my hair grow, and traded my starched shirt and black tie for a chambray shirt and bell-bottomed jeans. I spoke my mind about politics and social causes without fear of retribution. I felt liberated.

Ironically, my liberation had started with Sallie. When she appeared in my Athens office, I didn't know how to bridge my spirituality with my politics, my social values with my personal responsibilities. Sallie came and left in a whirlwind, leaving me unsettled and confused, but in her wake, I found my way. From my religious upbringing, I bring the core value of service to others. As a Unitarian, I value people of all beliefs. And as a feminist, I honor women who—like Sallie and so many others—know better than anyone else what is right for them and their families.

Coming into myself was a relief. I am grateful for the journey, but it was not without cost. In addition to losing Ben and my hometown community, I lost my marriage.

I had asked far too much of LaMerle, and I was no longer the conventional man she had married. In 1973, when the children were five, seven, and nine years old, we divorced. Leaving my children was the hardest thing I have ever done, and creating deeper relationships with Curtis Jr., Lori, and Kyle became more important to me than I had ever imagined. That deep commitment continues to this day. LaMerle later said that marrying me was the best thing that had happened to her and divorcing me was the second best. I hope she still feels that way. In the long run, I believe, it has proved the best outcome for all of us.

· · · ·

I continued to do abortions at my office in an old hacienda at the top of a hill on a dirt road named Camino Militar ("Military Road"). All patients were still referred through the CCS network, and the majority flew in from Texas. My devoted nurse, Reggie, who had moved to Santa Fe to continue our work, would meet each group at the airport in Albuquerque wearing her red scarf so they could identify her as their safe ride to my office. My hair was longer, and my workload was lighter. I saw my children more and had time for friends. I felt unburdened in more ways than I could name.

Then on January 22, 1973, the Supreme Court ruled on the case of *Roe v. Wade*. Abortion was now legal across the land.

Reggie and I were listening to the radio on that January day as we saw patients, awaiting what we believed would be an unfavorable ruling from the conservative court. When the news finally came, we were shocked: We had won! Reggie and I embraced as people did when the Spirit moved them in the churches of our East Texas childhood, bursting into tears of relief. Not only was I safe from prosecution, but the right to abortion was finally secure. Women would be safe and free from the shame and stigma of illegal abortion.

At last, it was over.

I was confident that most qualified doctors would provide abortions as a part of routine health care, and naturally I would be one of them. But before we could begin in earnest, I had one final task.

The ministers in Dallas called immediately after the Supreme Court decision, asking me to establish the first legal abortion clinic in Texas. Of course, I said, "Yes!"—with relief and enthusiasm this time. Within a month, I returned to Dallas. My former office was still available for lease, so I used that familiar space as a temporary clinic while I purchased a larger office down the street. The mortgage was arranged through the CCS ministers and guaranteed on my handshake.

Young doctors in residency programs in Dallas were eager for training, and young feminists were ready to work. I thought securing this clinic space would be quick and easy—my final contribution to the cause for which I'd risked so much. As I would have to learn again and again, things rarely go as expected.

CHAPTER TWO

Alone in the Dark: The Education of an Abortionist

*"I've made plenty of mistakes in my time
but I do not believe this is a mistake."
—Patient journal entry*

Curtis

As a child, I knew the women in my world had secrets. Men and women ruled different domains and, in many ways, led separate lives. They occupied opposite sides of the aisle in church. They ate separately at family dinners, the women at a second seating after first serving the men. I saw very little resentment of these separate and, by current standards, unequal roles. It was life as we knew it, as it had always been. Still, I had my priorities. If I wanted to hear a good story—possibly an X-rated one—I should stay out of sight but within earshot of the women.

As far as I was concerned, Mama Boyd was the keeper of all secrets. She was my father's mother and an important mother figure to me. In fact, she seemed to nurture half the county. Plus, she was our resident medical expert, although she had no formal education. Like many of her generation, she had lived through hard times. Her family had traveled westward by wagon train from Mississippi to East Texas to escape the Civil War; some in the area still called it the War of Northern Aggression. They farmed the land, lived simply, and relied on faith in God and good rainfall to get by.

Mama Boyd's formal education, such as it was, came to an end at age fourteen when she married Daddy Boyd. Soon after, she had the first of her ten pregnancies—seven children and three stillbirths. Trained not in school but through experience and in the company of other women, Mama Boyd became a lay midwife. In the absence of medical doctors, she and other midwives delivered most of the babies in the area. When she wasn't delivering babies, she dispensed folk remedies for everything from warts to croup.

During the winter months, between fall harvest and spring planting, Mama Boyd hosted the ladies' quilting bee at her house. Women gathered in her living room, stretched their works-in-progress across wooden frames suspended from her ceiling, threaded their needles, and set to work. Their eyes were on their stitches, not each other, and certainly not on me. If they ever noticed I was there, in the midst of their clatter and chatter, they'd soon forget. I'd sit quietly on the floor, half hidden behind the bureau, careful not to move a muscle—not even to go to the bathroom—lest I break my invisibility spell. I only peed on myself once.

After the pleasantries and sweet tea, the real conversation would commence. The women talked about births and miscarriages, sex and blood, and parts of the human body I had never heard of. Sometimes they could be catty, like the time they agreed that one newlywed in the community should be shunned because her baby was born one day too early. The verdict: she must have had sex before marriage. "A day's as good as a year!" declared Aunt Mattie.

Sometimes the conversation was more medical. That's when I would see not only my beloved grandmother, the sturdy Dutch woman with a ready smile and great sense of humor, but also Sister Pearl—her church name—an acknowledged Wise Woman in this circle of women and the larger community.

"Sister Pearl," a young woman might venture, peeking up from her stitches, "is there anything you can do to help bring on my period?" I was too young to understand what a period was, let alone why someone would want one. I was certainly too young and too male to know how to crack the women's code. Eventually, I figured out that women who did not have periods often had babies. But it would take me years more to learn what Mama Boyd did to hasten the return of "Aunt Flo."

By then, I was in medical school and slowly finding my way out of the dark—with less help from my medical training than you might imagine. In my day, women's symptoms were too often dismissed as "all in the head"—heart disease being the classic example—and consistently understudied. Virtually all research studies, if the goal was improved treatment, were conducted on White male subjects. But I was fascinated by the mysteries of the human body—not only male but female too.

· · · ·

As a young student at the University of Texas Southwestern Medical School, I listened in lecture halls as I had listened in my grandmother's living room: with rapt attention. I never lost my desire to discover new treatments and techniques—a trait that would come in handy later. In family medicine, I learned about everything from treating colic in infants to managing heart disease in adults. My fellow residents and I learned to care for pregnant women and deliver babies. Beyond that, however, women were largely ignored in medicine.

Women's complaints were often dismissed as "neurotic," and their symptoms were chronically dismissed. Of course, medical students did not learn to perform abortions. During our obstetrics-gynecology (OB-GYN) rotations, we did learn to perform D&Cs for the legions of women who came to the emergency room with unexplained uterine bleeding or incomplete miscarriages. In more detail, a D&C is a simple process of gently dilating the cervix, the natural opening from the vagina into the uterus, with a sterile rod (or series of rods of graduated diameter if greater dilation was needed) and then inserting a curette—a long, slender, spoon-like medical instrument—to scoop out the contents of the uterus. Later, when abortion became legal, these patients miraculously disappeared from our hospitals, revealing the truth: most of these cases of unexplained bleeding and incomplete miscarriage were illegal abortions. But at the time, we had no way to know unless the patients told us, and virtually all of them kept their secrets.

Looking back, it is impossible to determine just how many abortions were performed in the United States during the 1950s and '60s, the years when I was in school and then starting my practice. Some experts estimate there were as many as 1.2 million a year—and each year, somewhere between one thousand and five thousand women died from the procedure.[2] While this death rate is unacceptable given the proven safety of legal abortion, the statistics shed some light on how common illegal abortions were at the time and show that in spite of the health risks, they were far safer than many might believe.

Despite the horror stories that dominate our popular history of illegal abortions, most were not performed with coat hangers and knitting needles. Of course, untrained and unqualified people did attempt abortion with non-sterile instruments, and criminal syndicates in some big cities did exploit women financially and put them at medical risk. Perhaps even more dangerous, some women—too ashamed to let anyone know they were pregnant—took matters into their own hands. Some women did indeed drink turpentine, douche with bleach, or insert sharp objects into their own vagina. But such cases were as memorable as they were tragic because they were not common in our nation's emergency rooms.

In reality, many illegal abortions were performed by individuals with at least some medical training, including doctors like me and others organized under the CCS. Members of feminist groups like the Janes—an underground network of feminist abortion activists and lay providers—were trained by physicians to perform abortions and then passed their knowledge on to other lay providers. Additionally, some nurses and midwives provided abortions in their homes or private offices, and they cared about the women they served and generally used sterile techniques.

Nonphysician practitioners typically made no attempt to empty the uterus but only to disrupt the pregnancy by briefly inserting an instrument through the cervix and, essentially, stirring. The patient would be instructed to go home and wait for the cramping and bleeding that would expel the pregnancy. Most of these patients were early in their pregnancy, and the procedure went as expected, so we seldom saw them in the emergency room. The only people who knew about these uneventful abortions were likely the patients and their providers.

These patients usually got vague instructions for aftercare but a clear instruction in case of complications: Don't return to the abortionist.[3] Go straight to an ER. As a medical resident in the ER, I saw that these women typically came because they had more bleeding and pain than they had expected. We would diagnose this as an "incomplete spontaneous abortion" (the medical term for miscarriage), perform a simple D&C in the ER, and send the patient home on oral antibiotics. The few patients who were seriously ill when they arrived in the ER or who did not respond to our basic care were admitted to the hospital for critical care managed by more experienced doctors, with assistance from me and the other residents.

Once our basic medical training was over, most of my fellow residents wanted bigger challenges than uncomplicated D&Cs. I sought bigger challenges too but continued to perform D&Cs throughout my training. I felt drawn to these women in need—a pull that I neither questioned nor explored. The procedure held added appeal because it played to two of my strengths: manual dexterity and a visual imagination. Computer-aided technology such as ultrasound and MRI, which allows us to "see" soft tissue structures within the body, did not exist yet. D&Cs were "blind" procedures, which were rare in medicine at that time. Doing a successful D&C required sensitive hands combined with the ability to create a mental image of the three-dimensional uterine space in which I was operating. Relying solely on my sense of touch as I worked in the dark was its own challenge—and involved a skill set that would one day become invaluable to me.

In the ER, I learned that potentially fatal problems with abortion most often resulted from one of three complications: uncontrolled infection (the most common cause of abortion-related death); internal injury (more specifically, perforation of the uterus); or hemorrhage (a term for excessive blood loss). This knowledge would later guide my practice, alerting me to the dangers I must avoid—for my sake as well as the sake of my patients. With prompt medical care, however, these three major issues could be managed. The greatest complication in performing early abortions was, in fact, the secrecy.

Shame and stigma did as much to harm women as the illegal abortion itself. Seeking medical care after an abortion meant the woman had to reveal her secret, and this was a vital secret to keep. Obviously, she was complicit in a crime—something no woman wanted revealed. Yet, for women in this difficult position, two other secrets were equally worth guarding.

Prior to what we loosely refer to today as the sexual revolution, the rules for women were clear: Virginity was required before marriage. Motherhood was to be embraced after it. At the very least, the illusion of these feminine virtues had to be maintained. Violation of either norm—lost virginity or rejection of motherhood—brought private shame and public stigma. Rather than risk exposure, some women risked their lives by not seeking medical help.

In the 1960s, although Texas law required physicians to report a suspected abortion, most residents did not go out of their way to do so—even when we suspected. In part, our silence was born of the fraternal nature of medicine. We had heard of reputable doctors who provided abortions for their regular patients or as a favor to a friend or colleague. One forced confession from a patient, and that doctor's career would be over. Unless we believed the patient had suffered unnecessary injury, we simply did not pursue the matter.

Don't ask.

Don't tell.

I made the mistake of reporting an abortion only once, during my first year of residency. A woman arrived in the emergency room, bleeding heavily. On examination, I found a large tear to her cervix—clear evidence of an attempted illegal abortion. I sutured the tear, performed a D&C, and admitted her to the hospital for observation because she had lost a lot of blood. When I spoke to her privately, she admitted that she'd had an abortion. Since she had suffered a serious injury, I dutifully followed the written rules and reported it.

The next day, two policemen arrived at the hospital. As the medical resident who had made the report, I was summoned to the patient's room. The policemen questioned the patient, trying to get her to reveal the name of the abortionist. She refused. The detectives became more aggressive, even threatening her with jail.

I stood at the back of the room trying to distance myself from the scene, while the patient glared at me over the detectives' shoulders, as if saying, *How could you have done this to me?* I bowed my head; I'd had no idea the police would harass her. I thought they wanted the abortionist, not her. Yet they badgered her for what seemed hours.

Despite their threats, she admitted nothing. She remained steadfast, even defiant. After the detectives left, I went back to the patient's room to apologize and explain that I was in my first year of residency—that it was my first time reporting a suspected abortion and that it would be my last.

"The police will not bother you again," I assured her. Fortunately, they did not.

I was true to my word: I never reported another suspected abortion. I had violated an important trust and seen the consequences. Never again would I reveal a woman's secret.

. . . .

Practice is the best teacher, and with practice, I developed a system. In the early days in my Athens office, first-trimester abortions soon became routine. While the vast majority of these procedures went smoothly, a few did not. These complications became my real teachers.

Lesson one: prevent infection.

My work in the ER had taught me that abortion-related infection had two causes: non-sterile objects entering the uterus and pregnancy tissue not coming out. The risk of infection was greater in those days because lay providers only disrupted the pregnancy, and tissue retained in the uterus was a breeding ground for infection. On the other hand, doctors who quietly performed abortions in their office or hospital saw few infections because they used sterile techniques and, as I would soon learn, completely emptied the uterus.

The abortions these doctors provided were virtually identical to the D&Cs we'd trained to do as residents faced with all those incomplete miscarriages. Starting out in my own practice, I knew what to do. I planned for everything necessary to provide a safe abortion in my office—except general anesthesia. I couldn't safely put patients to sleep in my office. Some amount of discomfort would be unavoidable. For me, inflicting pain on patients has always been the most difficult part of practicing medicine.

The "blood and guts" aspect of medicine had never been a barrier for me. Growing up on a subsistence farm, we had slaughtered farm animals and wild game as a routine part of life. Despite being accustomed to bloodshed, I confess that I was caught off guard when I observed my first major abdominal surgery. Although the patient was under deep anesthesia, arteries were pulsing, and the rhythmic contractions of intestines continued. This motion, and the smell of antiseptics mingled with fresh blood as the surgeon swiftly clamped off the bleeding vessels, made the bright lights of the surgery room dance, and I swooned. Fortunately, a classmate caught me as I slumped toward the floor. At the time I was mortified, but I quickly desensitized to the necessary gore of surgery, grew to love the mysteries contained within the human body, and took pride in the manual dexterity surgery required.

However, I never adjusted to causing pain. Seeking to minimize abortion pain, I initially came too close to doing what the lay providers did: I would insert a sterile curette into the uterus and sweep its inner surface just enough to disrupt the pregnancy, hoping the sterility of my instrument and the dexterity with which I "stirred" would suffice.

However, two of my first patients ended up in emergency rooms with "incomplete miscarriages." I was increasing the health risk and hospital cost to my patients, not to mention the legal risk to me. My technique had to change.

Clearly, I had to perform a complete D&C for patients in my office, just as I had in the hospital, but without general anesthesia. By asking myself the right question—*What is stopping me from doing what I know is necessary?*—I shifted my focus to developing the most effective way to use a local anesthetic to block pain. If dentists could do it, surely I could too.

Adequate pain control, although short of my ideal, allowed me to thoroughly empty the uterus. No other patient suffered a serious infection in all my years of prelegal abortion.

. . . .

My next medical complication happened early in my first year of working with the CCS. By then, I had performed hundreds of first-trimester procedures in my office without problems. This particular complication occurred with a patient who was eleven weeks pregnant. I can't remember where she came from or how she got to Athens, but I will never forget the sinking feeling in the pit of my stomach when, as I finished her procedure, my instrument went deeper into her body than it should have.

Lesson two: avoid perforation.

I had pushed through the wall of her uterus and entered the abdominal cavity with its major blood vessels and bowels. And I was in there blind. I had no way of knowing how serious things could be, but I knew that if she bled excessively, I would have to hospitalize her—regardless of the consequences for me.

I observed the patient closely and was relieved when she remained stable and symptom free. At the end of the day, I released her with detailed instructions, antibiotics, and orders to call immediately if she felt faint or began to bleed. She did call, the following day.

"How are you feeling?" I asked.

"Fine," she replied, to my relief. "And grateful."

As perforations go, this one turned out to be minor. Back then, no one knew how common small uterine perforations are, particularly among rookie doctors, or that while some can be serious, even life threatening, most are minor and heal on their own. At the time, I only knew that my confidence was shaken. Things could have gone very badly.

Chastened by the experience, I reexamined my technique. I decided to dilate the cervix more so that I could evacuate the uterus faster, reasoning that the shrinking uterus would seal a small perforation. More dilation would increase the likelihood of a cervical injury, however, which left me with an additional problem to solve: To avoid damage to both the cervix and the uterus, I had to know where the tip of my instrument was at all times. I had to be both gentle and thorough—a difficult, but crucial, balance to strike.

I came to think of my curette as an antenna of sorts, what I would come to think of as my "feeler." I would hold the instrument lightly between my thumb and index finger, like a feather, and start by exploring the depth and shape of the cervix, then read the map of the uterine cavity. In this way, I could "see" in the dark.

I began the process of teaching myself with each patient by staying attentive and focused, noting every sensation—both my own and the patient's. Soon it became clear there were two of me: the "observing me" and the "doing me." I sent the observing me above the operating table to look over my shoulder and give constant feedback to the doing me. The observing me became my most helpful, and critical, teacher. I still teach young doctors to develop both a doing and an observing self so they can continually perfect their technique while staying attuned to the patient's needs and feelings.

Patients' reactions can provide valuable information, and attending to them humanizes the experience for both patient and doctor. It took me tens of thousands of patients to master this technique of observing while doing.

. . . .

By the time many women determined that they were pregnant and found the Clergy Consultation Service, they were already nine to twelve weeks along—approaching the limits of my experience. Since this was before the advent of ultrasound to visualize the pregnancy, and menstrual dates and pelvic exams are less reliable, there were surprises. For the most part, I handled these surprises by doing what I'd been trained to do and completing the task I'd begun. But the time came when I had to seek understanding beyond my training.

Lesson three: prevent hemorrhage.

I'd been taught that entering the pregnant uterus after twelve weeks carried a high risk of hemorrhage and even death, and in fact, the patient's medical risks do increase as the pregnancy develops. As the uterus stretches to accommodate the growing "fetal-placental unit" (the medical term), the uterine wall thins, and the blood supply to the uterus increases to support that growth. Additionally, at about eighteen weeks, the soft fetal bones begin to calcify. Thus as the fetal-placental unit grows larger and stronger, the uterus becomes more vulnerable to damage—increasing the risk of hemorrhage or a uterine tear. Additionally, since doctors had little to no experience terminating pregnancies after this point, they had no experience emptying the uterus quickly enough with only a curette. A healthy uterus shrinks as soon as it's empty, and the shrinking closes off the blood vessels, thus limiting bleeding.

Due to these increased risk factors, the medical community simply imposed a "Do Not Enter" rule. That rule went unquestioned. Medical students were taught that what happens in a pregnant woman's body is "natural" and thus not subject to the same level of scrutiny given injury or illness. If a woman needed to end a pregnancy after twelve weeks due to a serious medical problem—her own or with the fetus—the Do Not Enter rule obliged her to wait until she was sixteen weeks pregnant to be hospitalized for a medically necessary "termination of pregnancy" (TOP) by a physically and emotionally stressful method. She would be admitted to an obstetrical (OB) ward, where harmful medications would be injected into the pregnancy, and then given medication to stimulate uterine contractions until she delivered a dead fetus. These

TOP patients were typically ignored, if not shamed, by the OB nursing staff and by fellow patients. Women who needed to terminate a pregnancy were treated like failures—as mothers, as women, as members of society. It seems unthinkably cruel now, but that was the attitude in medicine and the community at the time.

Occasionally a woman would arrive in the ER with an incomplete second-trimester miscarriage. We medical residents had been taught that spontaneous abortions were common in the early weeks of pregnancy—current data and expert opinion place early pregnancy loss at about 30 percent—but far less common after twelve weeks.[4] In hindsight, many of these later "miscarriages" were probably failed attempts to abort the pregnancy, but we were clueless. We observed these women cramping as if in labor, and we hoped they would expel the pregnancy. If they did not, they bled heavily. Little was understood about managing miscarriages after twelve weeks, so none of us knew that removing both the pregnancy and the placenta attaching it to the uterus could stop the bleeding. In this case, ignoring the Do Not Enter rule could actually offer a cure.

In 1968, providing abortions alone in rural East Texas, I strayed into the forbidden twelve-week territory only by mistake. What I thought was an eleven-week pregnancy would turn out to be twelve. When I had made that error enough times and the procedures went smoothly, I set twelve weeks as my limit. Then, what I thought was a twelve-week pregnancy might actually be a thirteen- or even fourteen-week pregnancy. These procedures were technically more challenging, but I got consistently good results. Week by week, I worked my way into the second trimester. Soon I was doing abortions at sixteen weeks with relative ease.

Then I met Betty.

Unlike most of my patients, Betty was older, already in menopause—when periods become irregular, then cease altogether. By the time she and her doctor realized she had a menopausal pregnancy, she was nearly seventeen weeks pregnant and desperate. She was ready to be a grandmother, not a full-time mother all over again. I knew her own doctor had referred her to the CCS, so clearly, he supported her decision. I wanted to help her. So, buoyed by my previous successes, I pushed my limit.

I began the procedure as I would any other, but before I could remove the pregnancy, I had a basin full of blood—and more kept coming. I did what I could to slow the bleeding, with no success. This was a hemorrhage.

I knew it could be my downfall, but I had no choice. I called an ambulance and had her admitted to the Henderson County Memorial Hospital with a diagnosis of hemorrhage of unknown origin. Although the hospital was just across the street, the fact that I called an ambulance to get her there says it all: Betty was bleeding to death, and I was terrified.

I ordered transfusions. First one unit of blood, then a second, and still her bleeding did not stop. I ordered two more units STAT, only to learn they were the last two available units of her blood type. What if they didn't do the trick? I had to make a plan. The largest hospital in our area was thirty-five miles east, in Tyler, a town of fifty thousand. I called the OB-GYN in Tyler, whom I used for referrals, and put a hospital ambulance on alert.

The third unit went in, and Betty's bleeding continued.

I knew that when doctors in Tyler examined Betty, they would, of course, find that she was pregnant and realize this was a uterine hemorrhage with a known origin: I had attempted an abortion at seventeen weeks. My action was both illegal and a breach of accepted medical standards. Those thoughts flashed through my racing mind, but saving her life was my sole focus.

When I started the fourth transfusion in preparation for the ambulance trip, our fortunes turned. Betty stopped bleeding. I canceled the ambulance and let the doctor and hospital in Tyler know that she would not be coming.

Although Betty's bleeding had stopped, I knew that it could start again; I kept her in the hospital overnight. The next morning, she was stable, and we made a new plan. She wanted to go home to Dallas, and I could not finesse completing her abortion in Athens. She was to call her doctor, say she was having a miscarriage, and ask him to admit her to the Dallas hospital, where he could manage her care. She promised to call me as soon as she could with an update.

Two days later, Betty called. The news was good: she had expelled the pregnancy in the hospital without further problems. She was safe. And so was I, but a part of me—perhaps the observing me—wondered if my medical school professors had been right to hold the line at twelve weeks and I had simply been lucky. I needed to understand what had happened.

I replayed that procedure in an endless mental loop: What could I have done to cause such bleeding? What could I do to prevent it in the future? Was hemorrhage a normal occurrence at this stage of pregnancy, as I'd been taught, or was this an aberration? I was asking the right questions, but I had no answers. There were no experienced colleagues, much less experts, to consult. I was alone in my dilemma.

Hemorrhage is a life-threatening complication, and I could not risk a patient death. But I was only in my second year of performing illegal abortions, with no end in sight. Women would keep coming to me for help. How could I turn them away because they were a day, a week, or even several weeks into the second trimester, especially knowing what they had to go through just to get to my door? Despite what I'd overheard at Mama Boyd's quilting bees, a day further along in a pregnancy is not the same as a year. I knew I could not withhold care from all the women who were beyond the twelve-week mark.

But I made a promise to myself: I would wait for abortion to become legal before I would risk another abortion beyond sixteen weeks, and my observing self would pay even closer attention when performing the procedure for any patient between twelve and sixteen weeks.

Thus I paused in my slow process of pioneering a procedure known today as dilation and evacuation (D&E), which allows abortion providers to safely perform second-trimester abortions in outpatient facilities. In fact, the D&E is now performed through the second trimester.

Today, after fifty years of experience, I look back at my younger self and think my determination to create this better procedure was lunacy. Even knowing my ultimate success in creating a safer, more humane abortion experience for women, I question myself. Was I wise and compassionate—my preferred version of the story, naturally—or arrogant and foolhardy? I was already risking my career and freedom by performing abortions early in pregnancy, and abortion was illegal at any stage. What made me think this was the time for the risks inherent in developing any new surgical technique?

Back then, however, I felt I could rely on my more skillful version of the D&C up to sixteen weeks—but not beyond. For the time being, I had reached my limit. Even so, I sometimes failed to say no when I should have.

· · · ·

Saying yes was easy. I only needed to hear a woman's story, to know her struggle. How could I turn away from her need? Saying no was another matter. This inability or unwillingness to say no created the worst surgical complication of my illegal abortion career.

In 1969, soon after I learned the hard way that sixteen weeks was my limit, Reverend Claude Evans of the Clergy Consultation Service referred a patient to me: Lisa, a Southern Methodist University student. Reverend Evans didn't know, and I doubt Lisa realized either, that she was at least seventeen weeks pregnant—and I had just learned that sixteen weeks was my limit.

"I'm sorry," I told her, "but I can't help you."

Lisa burst into tears. As she pleaded, my heart ached for her, but I could not risk her health and life.

"I don't know how to safely do an abortion for you," I said.

She cried uncontrollably, repeating how desperate she was.

My resolve weakened, and I made a suggestion: "Call your doctor. If he will hospitalize you for a 'miscarriage,' I will start the process." Since I could not involve another physician in my illegal act, she left my office to make the call.

Thirty minutes later, Lisa returned saying she'd reached her doctor and told him that she was out of town and thought she was having a miscarriage. He had instructed her to return to Dallas so he could hospitalize her.

Violating my self-imposed sixteen-week limit—not to mention my professional decision to pursue medicine instead of religion—I proceeded on faith, inserting a curette into the uterine cavity and disrupting her pregnancy. She left for Dallas bleeding lightly and leaking amniotic fluid. Her abortion was inevitable. She could now have a "miscarriage" safely managed by her doctor in a Dallas hospital.

Two days later Reverend Evans called to tell me that Lisa had required an emergency hysterectomy. She had no doctor. She had lied to me.

I was shocked, and for a moment I felt betrayed. Then I recalled her desperation. Of course, she would have said anything to get me to do her abortion. She was ignorant of the risks to her life and health. I was the doctor, she had placed her trust in me, and I had failed her. Lisa was nineteen years old, and she would never be pregnant again. I was devastated.

"Curtis, you must learn to say no," Reverend Evans said. "You jeopardized the future."

I knew he was right. If I could not finish a procedure, I must not start it. Retained pregnancy tissue can lead to potentially fatal hemorrhage as well as infection. The big-city teaching hospitals, where I had once dreamed of having a career and which I held in such esteem, were no more capable of managing Lisa's abortion than I had been. I was alone in my work, and there was too much at stake to act on faith. This was medicine, not religion, and I had only myself to rely upon. No physician wants medical complications, but avoiding them was essential to my survival.

One of the goals of medical training is to learn from mistakes—preferably those of others. With abortion, I was working in isolation and had to learn exclusively from my own. Most of my complications occurred in the first four years—never, fortunately, more than two or three per thousand patients. As I acquired the necessary knowledge and enhanced my skill, my initial hospitalization rate of approximately one in one thousand patients quickly dropped to about one in five thousand. Between 1967 and 1973, I performed over fifty thousand abortions.

Revisiting these few cases still causes me pain, especially when I consider the irreparable damage I caused Lisa. I cannot undo my mistakes, but I learned valuable lessons. I find some measure of comfort in knowing that almost without fail, I recognized problems quickly and took action immediately. Being alert and nimble allowed me to contain many situations that could have developed into urgent complications. In many cases, the techniques I established in response to a complication are still used today by physicians all over the country.

When abortion became legal, I eagerly began to teach others so they could be spared my mistakes, and I believe my hard-earned humility has made me a better teacher.

. . . .

As I was performing Sallie's illegal abortion in my rural East Texas doctor's office in 1967, Colorado was legalizing abortion under certain circumstances—the first state in the union to do so. California, Oregon, and North Carolina quickly followed. In 1968 and '69, as I worked with the CCS and learned those painful lessons in how to provide more and safer abortions in my practice, six more states reformed their abortion laws.[5] The pendulum of history was beginning to swing in favor of women's health care.

The freedom that came with legalization enabled technological advances, and a vacuum aspirator designed specifically for abortion procedures became available in the United States. Having read reports of similar machines used in Russia, Eastern Europe, China, and ultimately the United Kingdom, I ordered one of the first vacuum aspirators made by Berkeley Bioengineering in California. Essentially a medical version of a household vacuum cleaner but with very gentle suction, the machine would be faster and more effective than doing the D&C by hand as I'd been taught. The tubing was designed to be sterilized between each use, and the suction cannulas came in sterile packaging from the manufacturer. The process would be safer too and cause less pain while also reducing the risk of infection, perforation, and bleeding. I could hardly wait to use it.

I was in a state of agitated excitement as I awaited delivery of the new machine to my office. I imagined that the police would somehow know the minute the shipment crossed the border into Texas, where abortion was still illegal, and show up at my door to arrest me for my crime. That did not happen, of course, but another horror story I had heard also concerned me.

In Colorado, where abortion was newly legal, some doctors using a standard surgical suction machine with reversible airflow had unintentionally blown air into the patient's uterus, resulting in her death. Even though the vacuum aspirator's airflow was not reversible, when my machine arrived, I stayed up half the night, taking it apart and putting it back together. Before using it on a patient, I needed to reassure myself that it would only vacuum.

The next day, my patients and I were rewarded. I could complete a first-trimester abortion in less than ten minutes. It's hard to overstate the positive impact this new technology had on my practice. In fact, it is hard to overstate the importance of all that I learned the hard way. I would later find that many doctors of conscience across the US had similar experiences. But at the time, most of us still worked in isolation—finding our own way, imagining that we alone had found the better way.

Change was coming faster and faster. With abortion becoming legal state by state, the Centers for Disease Control (CDC) formed the Abortion Surveillance System in 1969 to study legal abortion, the characteristics of women seeking abortion, and complication rates. Founded in 1946 as the Communicable Disease Center—the national public health agency of the United States—the CDC was initially charged with preventing the spread of malaria in the United States. Now, for the first time, abortion providers could voluntarily report complications—along with other relevant data—to the government. As soon as my work became legal, I was eager both to report to the CDC and to compare my experience with that of other providers. I welcomed the scientific community that came with governmental oversight. I was no longer alone.

So little was known about abortion when the CDC began its study, and so much was assumed. There were assumptions that abortion was dangerous, particularly in outpatient settings, and that abortions performed past twelve weeks of pregnancy were particularly so. However, by 2000, when Drs. Willard Cates Jr., David A. Grimes, and Kenneth F. Schulz published "Abortion Surveillance at CDC: Creating Public Health Light Out of Political Heat" in the *American Journal of Preventative Medicine*, they confirmed based on thirty years of study what I learned from my short years of very private practice:[6]

Suction curettage was safer than sharp curettage, local anesthesia was safer than general anesthesia, free-standing clinics were safer than hospitals, and dilation and evacuation (D&E) was safer than the alternative of labor induction for early second-trimester abortions. This evidence, which contradicted traditional medical tenets, rapidly changed the practice of abortion in the United States.

The CDC surveillance system also indicated "rapid improvement" in abortion safety starting in the early 1970s, with investigations of abortion-related deaths helping to transform practices. Data collected by the CDC offered pivotal insights into the abortion issue, often guiding judiciary and legislative decisions as well as reports by the surgeon general. With more data on abortion than any other operation in the history of medicine, the CDC's research supported safer reproductive choices for women. "When medical historians of the future look back on this century," the article claimed, "the increasing availability of safe, legal abortion will stand out as a public health triumph."

It would be gratifying if this story could end on such a vindicating note, but as we all know, that's not what happened. While abortion patients, providers, and advocates enjoyed a brief respite in the mid-1970s, the rise of the religious and political right would soon create a more hostile social climate than I ever experienced as an illegal abortionist.

CHAPTER THREE

Do Good Work: My Not-Quite-Accidental Career

"Today was the 1st day of a situation that almost stopped my heart.
My 14-year-old daughter was pregnant + when I found out she was
almost 7 months, I thought a spear went thru my heart, she was raped
and kept it to herself (she's my trooper). When she told me she
would rather kill herself than have a child I prayed to God to let me
get myself together and understand what was happening. I could write
forever but I won't. Thanks to the entire staff here that has given my
entire family a 2nd chance at life. This is a journey that we all have
went through together, everyone will always be in my heart. From a
mother who wouldn't give up on her baby girl, THANKS."
—*Patient journal entry*

Glenna

When Nathaniel Hawthorne wrote the classic novel *The Scarlet Letter* in
1850, the red letter *A* stood for adultery. Nearly two centuries later, the
A is for abortion, but the story is the same: women are shamed and cast

out for their sexuality while the men watch from the sidelines as if it's not their problem.

My long, not-quite-accidental career as an abortion counselor and abortion clinic owner has provided many opportunities to reflect on *The Scarlet Letter* and the power of shame and stigma, but Hawthorne holds a place of honor in my personal story for a different reason.

The scene is vivid in my memory. It's 1950, and I'm three years old, sitting on the living room floor with *The World Book Encyclopedia*—my third birthday gift. It's summer and Modesto, California, is "valley hot" outside, but the floor is cool, and I'm pulling those big books off the bookcase shelf. I'm in love with them: They take me to a larger world than the little brick house in the apricot orchard on the outskirts of town, where I live with my parents and my baby brother, Eddy. Since I can't yet read, I'm looking at pictures for the important people. I plan to be one too.

I'm the center of my own universe, so I already know how important I am. When I have a headache, I'm terrified because I think the whole world has it too, and I don't know how it can go on with such pain. But right now there's no headache, and I'm looking for pictures of girls, page after page, with no luck. Finally, in the *H* volume, I find her. She has a long name, and her hair is in fluffy curls, just like mine. Now I'm certain that I can have a place in the encyclopedia.

But when I show my mother, she begins an erudite lecture on men's hairstyles through the ages, starting with the Romans. Then she helps me sound out the encyclopedia girl's name: Nathaniel Hawthorne. Not a girl at all! Mother laughs, but I don't think it's funny.

· · · ·

My mother's brilliance in school was legendary in the family. She had skipped so many grades that she'd graduated from high school before her fifteenth birthday. Mother knew that children were smarter than the grown-ups thought, so throughout my own childhood, she made a point of never talking down to me or Eddy. She'd heard *You're not old enough to understand* far too many times from her own mother, and the memory still rankled.

Stories of my beloved mother's upbringing festered in my mind too, and from a very early age I hated my maternal grandmother. For starters, Nama believed children should be seen only rarely—and never heard. But for me, the unforgivable thing was her contempt for my father, who—as a Norwegian immigrant—was somehow part of a servant class. My grandmother never allowed Daddy to sleep in her home, instead booking a hotel room for him. On one of our annual visits to Nama, I walked into her bedroom, hoping to play in the jewelry box on her dressing table. Instead, I found my mother seated at the dressing table in tears as Nama berated her for following her heart and "marrying beneath her station in life." I quietly backed out of the room and knew, at age eight or nine, that I truly despised the witch.

Mother had grown up wanting to be a doctor, but my grandmother quashed that dream too. Years later—as a student myself, pursuing a degree in psychology—I would come to appreciate B. F. Skinner, the behavioral psychologist, for the opening line of his autobiography, which I have always remembered as "My grandmother was a social climber."[7] So was mine. I would also come to understand my mother's compassion for Nama, a woman who was deeply damaged by life.

By then, I had long known that I was both a joy and a burden to my mother and that parenthood should be undertaken with full knowledge of the sacrifices required. To me, it makes perfect sense that the majority of abortion patients I see already have at least one child. They know from experience the responsibilities of motherhood, and they want to do their best for their families—even if what is best requires a difficult, sometimes unthinkable choice.

My own path led away from a career as a medical doctor because I imagined that I would be stealing my mother's dream. Yet I eventually found my way to a very special field of medicine, entering abortion care and becoming a doctor of psychology—not to mention marrying a physician. I found my way to a lifetime of doing something important.

My career is no accident.

. . . .

Right before I started kindergarten, we moved from our little house in the country to a California Craftsman cottage on a paved street inside the city limits. I thought the move was a bad idea, and so did Smokey, my cat. She hid under the sofa for at least a week. Daddy and I worried that Smokey would run away. Daddy had grown up on a farm in a Norwegian immigrant community in South Dakota and understood the ways of animals and children. He explained that Smokey missed her home in the countryside as much as I did, but he and Mother wanted me to go to the best school, and it was not on the outskirts of town.

Smokey and I adjusted, but I missed our long walks in the orchards blooming with apricots, peaches, and cherries. Heaven. Plus my first pet, Timmy, a surprisingly affectionate canary, was buried under one of the apricot trees. Mother got Timmy while she was pregnant with me. She told me that he would sit on her swollen belly and sing to her when she'd had to rest late in her pregnancy. I thought of Timmy as the spirit of her pregnancy—me before I was me—and I loved him. He would sing for hours and perch on my finger, pecking my cheek as if giving me a kiss.

When I was going on three and Mother was pregnant with Eddy, Timmy got very sick. A neighbor told my parents to give him a teaspoon of whiskey in an eyedropper as a merciful way to let him die. But he lingered, and Daddy finally took him outside and, like the good farm boy, snapped his tiny neck. Mother held me in her arms, and I cried so hard I couldn't breathe. Then Daddy came back inside, and we all cried together. Mother wrapped Timmy in tissue paper, and I got my favorite shoebox—it was from my very first pair of patent leather shoes, so I kept precious things in it—and we placed Timmy inside and buried him beneath my favorite apricot tree.

Dead or not, I thought it was wrong to leave Timmy behind when we moved to the city. And I thought Mother missed him too, because I'd catch her with a faraway look in her eyes, and when she saw me, she'd sometimes wipe tears from her cheeks. I had thought she only cried when I was sad. Now I could see that she went to a sad place of her own. But I didn't have time to solve the mystery of my mother because just as she and Daddy had planned, kindergarten started, and it was more wonderful than I could have imagined, with so many new friends and recess and the jungle gym. Maybe my parents had been right to move, and everything would be fine.

Then I came home from school one day in first grade to find Mother sitting at the kitchen table—pearl-gray Formica with a chrome wrap-around and chairs to match. The lights were off, and in my mind, I can still see her in the shaft of daylight from the window above the sink. She was backlit and beautiful, but she had gone to her sad place. I slipped behind her chair and put my arms around her shoulders, waiting for her to return to the room, to the present, and to me. I gathered my courage and asked, "What have I done wrong?"

Mother wiped the tears from her cheeks and took me in her arms, explaining that I'd done nothing wrong. "I'm sad because it's my father's birthday," she said.

That made no sense. His birthday should be a happy day, and I told her so. I needed to set her straight so she would stop going to the sad place. Instead, she told me a story I didn't want to hear: her father had committed suicide when she was a girl. "Suicide" was a new word for me, and I loved Mother's word games. But when she told me it meant he'd killed himself and she still missed him, I didn't like her new game. It made my tummy hurt, so I climbed into her lap and made her rock me—or maybe I was rocking her—and we both cried. Her sad place scared me, and now I knew why: parents died there.

Soon I would learn that my mother had another reason for her sadness, and it had to do with something else that had died when she was a girl: her dream of being a doctor. Unlike my new friends' mothers, who seemed satisfied to cook and clean and sew, Mother wasn't designed to be a happy homemaker. I envied those friends sometimes—not that I knew the word "envy," but I knew the feeling, especially after a fried chicken dinner at Cynthia Gregory's house. When I raved about it, I learned that Mother disapproved of all things fried.

But having a different kind of mother had its perks. She frequently took me out of school for educational field trips of her own design. We visited historic sites and museums, observed the migration of Canada geese at the bird refuge, and walked the windswept beaches at Point Lobos. I loved those trips and the unapologetic notes Mother wrote my teachers: *Please excuse Glenna's absence. The Paul Klee exhibit at the Armory Center for the Arts is remarkable, and it was important that she see it.* Her rebellious streak and her clear priorities—spending time in nature and exploring the work of great artists—are gifts I treasure to this day.

But one day in second grade I came home, and Mother wasn't there. I put on my roller skates and took off. I could almost fly on those skates, but my flight lasted only until dusk. When I returned, Mother's car was not in the driveway or the garage. I stood at the living room window, strumming the slats of the venetian blinds with my index finger, watching for her headlights. There was dust on the slats, and my head throbbed. My vision blurred. Finally, I saw the car lights and heard the familiar motor in the driveway. Mother was alive, and I could breathe again.

When she came in, though, her face was splotched and her eyes were red. She went straight to bed. I have no memory of Eddy or my father that night, although Daddy must have been home, quietly preparing dinner as he often did. I only remember feeling alone.

Later that week, Mother and Daddy called a family meeting. We gathered in the living room. Eddy and I sat on the sofa; Mother and Daddy brought in dining chairs so they could sit close to each other. We'd never had a family meeting, so I had no idea what was coming. Mother started by asking us what we really wanted, and I spoke right up. I knew what I wanted: a carriage for my baby doll, and I knew she'd get it for me.

Instead she seemed to completely change the subject. In keeping with her habit of honesty with children, she told us that when she'd disappeared the other day, her plan had been to drive headlong into an oncoming truck. Highway 99 ran the length of California, and in rural areas the huge semitrucks traveled at full speed. As she drove, however, she imagined Eddy and Daddy and me without her, and the truck drivers with families of their own, and she'd realized her plan was bad. She'd come home to us in utter despair.

"Utter despair" are the words I remember. I didn't understand those words, but her sad face and the catch in her throat told me enough. Too much, really.

Daddy held Mother's hand as she explained that she loved us beyond words and wanted to be our mother, but she could no longer spend her days keeping house or playing bridge and presiding over PTA meetings. So, she and Daddy had created a better plan: Mother would go to work when Eddy started school the following year. Daddy would say no to the promotion he'd been offered, which would have required us to move again. He would complete college, which he'd begun when I started kindergarten, and then start a business of his own. We would all be OK.

The honesty with which my parents faced the situation as a team with a problem to solve shapes and sustains me to this day. Somehow, in the midst of the 1950s, they recognized that my mother was not the problem, that the rigid roles so ingrained in society could be a silent killer. Years later, when I gave her a copy of *The Feminine Mystique*, Mother echoed her remarks at the family meeting: she had loved being a mother but found the role of 1950s homemaker and the prospect of also performing corporate wife duties intolerable. As usual, she spoke the truth.

Despite her prim and proper upbringing, my mother was anything but conventional. And although Eddy and I were both planned pregnancies, Mother was not domestic. Despite my early envy of friends whose mothers loved to cook and sew, by high school I knew that some of my classmates' mothers were closet alcoholics, and one friend's perfect '50s mother committed suicide in our senior year. My mother, with the full support of my father, saved her own life, but too many others did not. My story is not tragic; it's a story of tragedy averted.

With my parents' plan decided, I crawled into bed after the family meeting, my mind and stomach spinning with too many feelings. *What do you really want?* had been a trick question, which made me mad. But I was even more mad about giving the wrong answer. Babies in carriages would never be on my wish list now, and life as a homemaker was out too. What I wanted, most of all, was to protect my mother from herself.

That I'd taken up an impossible task was beside the point. At age seven, I had no clear sense of the limit of my powers. I needed to believe that I could do something to help.

. . . .

Although she returned to work, my mother did not have the career of her dreams. When my grandmother had refused to pay for Mother to attend medical school and threatened to disinherit her if she did anything so unbecoming to a lady, my mother's reaction had been decisive. At the age of twenty, she packed three trunks and moved from Coral Gables, Florida, to California to create a life on her own terms.

Mother selected California because it was far away from her mother and her privileged yet troubled childhood, and because dear friends from Florida had moved there and invited her to join them. Those friends later became my Aunt Gustie and Uncle Jack—my favorite relatives. Aunt Gustie was one of my father's five older sisters, and her husband, Jack, was a wonderful storyteller. Daddy and Jack entertained me throughout my childhood with stories of their youthful adventures—including riding a freight train with the hobos to buy their first car in Detroit. During the Great Depression, they drove that car to California, where my father, like so many migrants, could earn cash to send to his parents in a futile attempt to save their farm from creditors. Along the road, every tire on the car blew out. Each time, Daddy and Jack found day labor until they had enough money to buy a new tire. It was a long, slow trip to the promised land.

Eight years later, my mother traveled to California by train in the comparative luxury of a private sleeper compartment. The greatest hardship of her trip was going to bed somewhere in East Texas and waking the next morning—still in Texas. When Mary finally arrived at the quaint train station in Modesto, her friends sent a shy, handsome young man to meet her at the station: Gustie's brother Glenn. For my father, it was love at first sight.

At nearly six feet tall, Mary was strikingly beautiful and brilliant—in his eyes, an exotic creature from another world. I don't think my mother did "love at first sight." Her critical mind was always at work, and she was not looking for love. My father's gentle Scandinavian manner, however, was reminiscent of the Swedish nanny who had raised her. In his presence, she must have felt an immediate comfort.

Mother found work in Modesto as an office nurse for a respected doctor who willingly trained her to assist him with routine office procedures and whom I would later know as a trusted family friend until his death. Although she developed a close friendship with Glenn, she dated other men. My father told me about one rival: a tall, dark, and handsome man who was an excellent ballroom dancer. Glenn had worried until Mary reported that she'd seen the other man behave rudely to his own mother—not a gentleman! Glenn would not lose her to the fancy dancer.

They married when my father, a pacifist, enlisted in the US Army during World War II. Having learned of Nazi atrocities, he felt compelled to do his part. He spent the war in Australia and then in New Guinea running a supply depot. My childhood home was filled with art and artifacts from New Guinea, including photos of my blond Norwegian father surrounded by the native people he had befriended: women in grass skirts with breasts that seemed to hang to their knees. I was entranced. My mother was more interested in his humanitarian values.

After our family meeting and around the time I started third grade, Mother returned to work to cure her depression and again found a job with a respected physician. She did her best, juggling child-rearing with her career as an office nurse, because life would have been incomplete without both. I remember the medical journals stacked by her bedside. If Eddy or I were so foolish as to watch *Ben Casey* or *Dr. Kildare* on TV, she'd sweep through the room with a stream of editorial comments, correcting those imposters as she went.

I always knew that her career was a compromise at best, but a life-saving one. It took me years to grasp the sacrifice my father made, especially at a time when men were measured solely by their career success—their role as the family breadwinner. Even then, though, I knew that we were his first priority. Daddy was the one who got me to school on time and took me for ballet lessons, the one who sat at my bedside reading *Little House on the Prairie* aloud when I had measles, and then *Little House in the Big Woods* with chickenpox. I was safe in his care.

I took the notion of equality between the sexes for granted because that's how it was at my house, but I also knew my parents neither expected nor valued convention. Hard work was far more important to them.

My father was still mastering the finer points of the English language when I was in grammar school. He'd worked his way up from bag boy to manager of what became the first supermarket in Modesto: Lucky Stores, with its tall, yellow marquee perforated with three squares for the three meals of the day. When he left Lucky to finish school, he continued to work full time. In exchange for his "better plan" with my mother, he had passed up the opportunity to become part of the management team that established the first chain of supermarkets in Northern California.

Although my mother considered herself an escapee from privilege and convention, her sense of decorum would dog her, and therefore me, to the end. Every morning as I left for grammar school, she covered the essentials, starting with "Do you have a clean handkerchief?" She might have rejected her mother's standards, but ladylike behavior was still required. That question was always followed by the equally important injunction "Do good work!" This meant at least two things: I was expected to excel in school and also to do good deeds in the world. Coming from my mother, there was an element of noblesse oblige. I had advantages and therefore a duty to help those who had less than I did.

In my childhood fantasies, I was a doctor on the SS *HOPE*, otherwise known as the Good Ship *HOPE*, ministering to the needs of exotic people in foreign lands. I was in seventh grade when the international health and humanitarian organization Project HOPE (Health

Opportunities for People Everywhere) launched its first voyage—to Indonesia and South Vietnam—and I was enchanted by the newsreel coverage and magazine photos. Project HOPE embodied the idealism of post–World War II America. The nation had emerged from the war on the winning side, as the acknowledged dominant global power with a strong enough economy to take my mother's charge to heart: Do good work in the world. I was inspired—plus devotion to such goals meant I could get out of Modesto and see the world.

In high school, I began taking aptitude tests and SATs, visiting colleges, and pondering my own options. As a young woman in the mid-1960s, I would have far more opportunities than my mother had in the late 1930s, as well as my parents' unconditional support. One thing I didn't have yet, though, was any idea what I wanted to do with my life.

. . . .

In my junior year of high school, 1964, President Lyndon Johnson declared war on poverty and established Title I funding for designated "poverty schools." The following year, I volunteered as an afterschool playground supervisor at the poverty school in South Modesto. The students were mostly poor White kids and a few children of Mexican farm laborers who'd managed to find year-round work. The job was fun: I was part playmate, part referee—a perfect fit for my bossy nature and athletic body. It was also my first experience with people from a world entirely unlike my own.

My need to enlarge my worldview continued throughout college, as did my need to do good work. While at Occidental College, I did volunteer tutoring for underprivileged children in Los Angeles and changed my major back and forth: sociology, psychology, English literature. I couldn't settle on just one and couldn't see a career that would fit my seemingly disparate interests.

By 1969, as a college senior, I was working as a teaching assistant for both my abnormal psychology professor and two teachers in the English department at East Los Angeles City College. At City College, I taught basic writing skills to students who'd failed the English competency exam. They were invariably older than I was and had life experiences far beyond my sheltered world. Each week they wrote a one-page essay about something in their lives, from how they came to live in LA to what they did at work. As I dutifully corrected grammar and punctuation, those essays sometimes brought me to tears and taught me that everyone has stories to tell—stories that deserve our attention.

One Sunday morning, the two City College teachers invited me for coffee at their home, a simple bungalow in an old LA neighborhood. They were the first openly lesbian couple I had known—others were "closeted," or tried to be—and I liked them. We sat in their atrium with warm sunlight filtering through a virtual forest of well-tended plants. The teachers praised my work: I was conscientious about punctuation, and my marginal comments were often insightful. They knew I cared about their students. Next to my coffee cup, however, they'd placed a box of No. 2 pencils and a sharpener.

The teachers asked me to forgo my red pen when grading the students' work so they could erase anything that would discourage students struggling to express themselves. When they pointed out my insensitive comments—*Cliché!* or *Awkward wording! Revise*—I struggled not to cry. They were right, and it was a lesson I never forgot. Those two women showed me how to deliver direct criticism with tact and kindness.

My attitude toward homosexual unions had begun to form in kindergarten when I fell in love with several of my new classmates—one boy and two girls. Although I slept with my boyfriend at nap time, our towels side by side as we chewed our fingernails in unison, I'd decided that I would marry one of the girls. They were prettier, and I wanted pretty children.

"Which girl should I marry?" I asked, trying to discuss this dilemma with Mother. When she laughed, that settled it. I'd show her: I'd marry them both plus the boy.

At that, I got another one of my mother's thorough lectures—this time on the legal status of polygamy in America. But Mother also assured me that I could wait before deciding. The important thing was to marry someone I loved.

Despite my mother's good advice and my stubborn unconventional streak, when I graduated from college, I took refuge in convention and did exactly what was expected of girls at the time: I married my college boyfriend, Rob.

My reasons were self-serving and partly hidden, even from myself. Rob had many virtues, intelligence being near the top of the list, and indeed that was important to me. But I knew, before we'd even said our vows, that our relationship was past its expiration date. His open disapproval of my visits with the lesbian couple should have been one of many clues that he wasn't "the one."

We moved from California to Texas—first Austin and then Dallas, where Rob had been admitted to a doctoral program in psychology embedded in the psychiatry department of the University of Texas Southwestern Medical School. With help from my parents, I supported Rob through his graduate training, deferring my own further education in favor of my first real job: counselor at a halfway house for chronic schizophrenics. I didn't know it yet, but going to work in the real world, learning that I was good at something other than school, and experiencing the satisfaction of being part of a work team would become the stars by which I would chart my professional life.

In part, I planned to let Rob test this unusual psychology program with an eye to submitting my own application if it proved worthwhile. I was also buying time to sort out my conflict between a love of literature and my fascination with psychology—between the lure of beautifully constructed imaginary worlds and the desire to change the real one. Although the marriage bought me time, both Rob and I paid an emotional price.

In the first year of our marriage, I had a pregnancy scare. The doctor at the student health center where I could receive free medical care decided it was time for me to take a break from the birth control pill. I'd been on it for over four years, and a hiatus was standard medical practice in 1970. Rob and I reverted to condoms and spermicidal foam. As the doctor had predicted, I had no menstrual period for several months. After the third or fourth month, I began to worry.

Home pregnancy tests did not yet exist, so I saw a private OB-GYN for a pregnancy test. The following day I got a call at work from the doctor's office. "Congratulations, honey!" said the nurse. "You're going to have a baby."

I burst into tears. Then I called a friend, who promised me the money to go to Mexico City for an abortion.

When I told Rob that I was pregnant, his response was adamant: "If you're pregnant, you're on your own. No way I'll support a child." I assured him that I'd already secured money for an abortion, but instead of the relief I'd expected, he yelled, "How dare you kill a baby of mine!"

My mind said, *You can't have it both ways.* My heart told me the marriage was over.

The next day, my very late and very heavy menstrual period began. In hindsight, I recognize that this was probably an early spontaneous abortion. My body, as well as my mind, was done with Rob.

No one in my family had ever divorced, so the deed was unimaginable. Despite the fact that by 1970 roughly half of all marriages in the United States would end in divorce, it carried a stigma I could not face and a sense of personal failure I could not accept.[8] Looking back, I find it ironic that I wasn't able to take comfort in the statistic. I see the same stigma-driven sense of personal failure in so many abortion patients despite my attempts to reassure them. During my career, roughly one in three US women has had an abortion at some point in her life, yet I have never met a patient who takes comfort in that statistic—just as the frequency of divorce was no comfort to me.[9] I felt alone in my predicament and kept my "failure" secret far too long.

It would take me four more years to actually divorce him. As I marked those lonely years, I devoted myself to work, learning from excellent colleagues and friendships that could sustain me. Our marriage became a series of separations and reconciliations. I was finding my professional direction but lost in my personal life.

. . . .

My first real job in Texas, at Turtle Creek Manor halfway house, seemed to incorporate the idealistic goals of the Community Mental Health Act signed into law during John F. Kennedy's presidency: to move patients out of the back wards of state mental hospitals into the community where they could, with our daily help, become functioning members of society. I was fascinated by the residents, many of whom had been written off by their families and society. Their words and actions might have seemed off-the-wall, but I often found meaning in the apparent madness. With guidance from skilled supervisors, I learned to listen closely, observe with care, and treat people with respect and dignity. Turtle Creek Manor had enough success to justify support from a state agency and private charities. Influential members of the Dallas community served on the board of directors, often drawn to the cause because someone in their family suffered from mental illness.

In my three years at Turtle Creek Manor, two residents became pregnant, one in 1970 and the other in 1971. The halfway house was their home, providing a semi-structured environment with regular meals, the socialization of group living, and regular individual and group therapy sessions. Residents were not confined within its walls, and most worked at odd jobs or sought training in sheltered workshops. We were responsible for keeping them on the antipsychotic medications of the time, which often blunted their emotions and caused other miserable side effects. This required monitoring by the full staff but freed the residents to be out and about in the community, which is the goal of any halfway house.

Given the freedom of the halfway house, many of the residents were no doubt sexually active, and the women were thus vulnerable to unintended pregnancies—with potentially disastrous consequences. Not only were many of these women unprepared to take on the responsibilities of parenthood, but the same medications that controlled their psychoses could cause serious damage to a developing pregnancy. These women were desperate to *not be pregnant*.

I had no doubt that abortion was a moral good. Growing up, abortion simply never entered my mind: it was neither a topic of conversation nor of controversy. I first saw the word as a fifteen-year-old, in the headline of a front-page story in the *Modesto Bee* above a photo of children's TV personality Sherri Chessen deplaning in Arizona after traveling to Sweden for an abortion. I asked my mother what "abortion" meant.

"It's a medical procedure to end a pregnancy that wasn't meant to be," she replied. "Meant to be" was one of her stock phrases, akin to "God's will" without invoking a god. Mother explained, with her usual thoroughness and accuracy, that Chessen had been taking the common sedative thalidomide, which had caused thousands of serious fetal malformations. I concluded that abortion was necessary medical care that allowed parents to avert tragedy, for themselves and their children.

Yet despite the need, abortion was illegal in Texas, as I knew all too well from my own pregnancy scare. I wasn't sure what I could do for the pregnant patients at Turtle Creek Manor, so I sought counsel from a judge who served on the board. He referred me to the chaplain at SMU: Claude Evans of the Clergy Consultation Service, who, in turn, referred me to Dr. Curtis Boyd.

Dr. Boyd's office, I discovered in 1970, was just five blocks from the halfway house. In spite of the chaplain's glowing recommendation of Dr. Boyd as well trained, ethical, and kind, I reasoned that a local MD performing illegal abortions literally down the street was probably disreputable. So I raised money from board members, bought airline tickets, drove the pregnant woman to the Dallas Love Field Airport, and saw her safely on her flight to Los Angeles, where abortion was legal and she could receive care at the Feminist Women's Health Center (FWHC).

The young woman had no wish to be pregnant, and the procedure went well, but the stress of travel was too much. When I met her return flight, a stewardess was helping her from the plane to the arrival lounge as she raved incoherently. I felt awful: I'd made a bad decision. Motivated by my own prejudices—in favor of abortion but mistrustful of abortionists—I had stressed an already vulnerable woman beyond her breaking point.

When the second resident needed an abortion, I was ready to risk the doctor down the street. But by then he'd relocated to New Mexico. So, once again, I sent a woman to Los Angeles, and once again, I saw that the difficulty of obtaining an abortion could cause far more trauma than the decision or the procedure. Travel to another, often distant, state was onerous; medical follow-up was unavailable; and the fact that the abortion was a crime in their home state sent a clear message to the women: *You are doing something wrong!*

Both women ultimately recovered, and I learned that access to abortion is critical to the physical and emotional outcome—a painfully real issue to this day. At the same time, I learned that judges and ministers saw the need for abortion, which reinforced my belief that abortion should be a legal right and is surely a moral good.

Given the holy war that now dominates the issue, it may seem strange that I didn't think about abortion in religious terms, but abortion was not yet cast as a religious issue in popular American culture. Support for birth control and abortion was as strong among Republicans of that era as it was among Democrats, with most preferring to remain silent on such private matters. When the feminist movement rose to prominence in the 1960s, the language in support of abortion had necessarily focused on the "legal right," and many mainstream American churches supported the cause. In fact, the strongest institutional support for legalization came from mainline Protestant churches, with the United Methodist, Presbyterian, United Baptist and Southern Baptist (who have since reversed their position), Unitarian Universalist, and United Church of Christ all writing formal position papers in support of legal abortion.[10]

After I had worked at Turtle Creek Manor for three years, the director of the halfway house moved to England to set up similar homes, and I searched for a new job. I had no plan, but Dallas was under a Supreme Court order to desegregate its public schools, and the Dallas Urban League—which had a number of federal grants to implement the court order—advertised for an educational counselor. The position seemed ideal. I'd been raised to believe in racial equality and saw civil rights as the most important issue of the time.

Here was my chance to do more good work.

· · · ·

Early in my tenure with the Urban League, I visited the all-Black high school I was to work with and observed two classes for students who read at or below a third-grade level. Thinking I could be useful as a teaching assistant, I got permission from the Urban League to dedicate part of my work time to teaching—if the White school principal would agree. He had not been receptive to my colleagues, but I thought the fact that I was White might prove an advantage.

I remember dressing conservatively for the meeting, making my pitch, and then meeting the principal's gaze as he said, "We all know the only reason a White girl comes into a Black neighborhood. It's to get fucked."

I was speechless in my outrage. His words were a clear dismissal, but I didn't move. When I found my voice, it was ice. "Do I have your permission or not?"

I got a parking pass and a laminated ID card that allowed me into the school. I never saw nor spoke to the principal again.

After a year and a half, I quit the Urban League. The White schools didn't want Black students, and those students didn't really want to be bussed into alien, often hostile White territory. It was a no-win situation. Even though I sensed that the problem was bigger than me, I took the defeat personally. Years later, I know that my work with school desegregation forever changed my understanding of the deeply embedded nature of racism in America, but at the time I was demoralized. I needed a change, and because I'm White and well educated, I could move on.

I needed to work for a "just cause," but I also badly needed a win. It was January 1974, one year after the Supreme Court had ruled in *Roe v. Wade* that abortion was legal throughout the nation. A friend who was working at the Fairmount Center, the first legal abortion clinic in Texas, told me they were looking for a counselor. The prospect of working for women, with women, was irresistible. Working for a social cause that had won a stunning victory seemed not only meaningful but easy in contrast to my experience at the Urban League.

In hindsight, my experience with the insidious resistance to school desegregation could have been a warning: sexism, like racism, is deeply entrenched in the history of the world and in American society—something even a Supreme Court decision cannot readily change. But I lacked such perspective. At the time, abortion seemed so straightforward.

I applied for the position based on my experience with those two residents of the halfway house and my confidence that I could do anything I set my mind to. When I showed up for my job interview, I noticed that the sign in the front yard read simply 2921 Fairmount. On a separate plaque below the address was the name Curtis Boyd, MD.

I was so intent on acing the job interview, I didn't think about the doctor's name. I was hired on the spot by an administrator who happened to be married to a classmate of my soon-to-be ex-husband, Rob. When I gave my two-week notice at the Urban League, they offered me a promotion, but I'd already made my choice.

My first day on the new job, I studied the Patient Medical History form and the Counseling and Procedure Progress notes to be completed by both counselor and doctor. That's when I registered the name that the letterhead bore: Curtis Boyd, MD. Although I had yet to meet him, I now worked for the same doctor I'd refused to refer patients to three years earlier.

My training consisted of observing the administrator as she counseled and then assisted in the abortion procedure with several patients. Although I liked the administrator, I was confident after my "training" that she knew even less than I did about what abortion counseling could be. My obvious lack of qualifications ceased to worry me. In truth, legal abortion was a new field, and no one knew what abortion counseling should be—or could be. I would need to create my own version, essentially from scratch.

I knew a bit about the feminist approach because I came of age in the midst of the feminist revolution of the 1960s and early 1970s. *Our Bodies, Ourselves*, the self-help manual that would become the classic feminist guide to women's sexuality and reproductive health, was published in 1970 and served as my bible. In 1971, when I facilitated a consciousness-raising group sponsored by Women for Change (the precursor to the Dallas Women's Center), I learned that feminist women's groups were explicitly not psychotherapy. Instead, I was told that we met to identify the ways we were oppressed by men and society. Our goal was to throw off our shackles and change the world—as if it would be that simple.

Having sent those two halfway-house residents to the Feminist Women's Health Center in Los Angeles, I knew the FWHC approach was also frankly opposed to counseling—I had provided the only counseling those women got.

I would have to look elsewhere for guidance.

I picked through files in the clinic's front office, where I found a manila folder labeled *Clergy Consultation Service* containing a single sheet of paper: "Guide to Counseling in Problem Pregnancy."[11] The first paragraph cast abortion as "the lesser sin" in the face of a problem pregnancy. In my worldview, abortion was both a moral and a social good. Despite the kindness I'd experienced with the SMU ministers, I decided the CCS approach would be no help either.

However, the same week that I dismissed the CCS guidelines, I counseled a pregnant college student. I liked her. During our pre-abortion meeting, I predicted she would do well with the procedure. She was physically healthy, seemed emotionally stable, and had the support of her boyfriend and parents. I held her hand as she lay on the exam table, gowned and prepped for her abortion. The physician inserted the suction cannula and turned on the vacuum aspirator. At the sound of the motor, the young woman's eyes grew wide. With an urgency that startled me, she blurted, "Will my baby go to hell?"

My answer was immediate and bypassed rational thought. "No! Of course not. God would never do that to an innocent being . . . nor to you."

As those words flew from my mouth, I knew two things: I would need to explore each patient's religious or spiritual beliefs before the procedure, and doing so would require ongoing attention to my own beliefs.

. . . .

My parents had intentionally omitted religious training from my childhood. My mother described herself as an agnostic, while my father told me that he'd been frightened by the hellfire-and-damnation sermons at the tiny Norwegian Lutheran Church of his childhood. Images of devils with pitchforks—a farm implement he had used daily—served as background for his firm belief that most evil in the world is perpetrated in the name of one religion or another.

I was four the only time my parents took me to church. We were there for the wedding of Jenny, the "big girl" next door to our house in the country. I thought the church was beautiful, with its paintings of white lambs in fields of green. If there was a nearly naked man being tortured on a cross, I didn't notice. I was busy looking at all the strangers in fancy clothes, especially when a girl only a little bigger than me started throwing white rose petals on the floor. Jenny, the neighbor girl, and her father walked behind the little girl and disappeared. When Mother wouldn't let me stand up on the hardwood bench to see better, I got bored. What did "wedding" mean anyway? What Mother explained sounded like a bad idea: Jenny was going to live with the man I hadn't seen and not have any more boyfriends for the rest of her life. Finally, we got to the part with cake, but it wasn't even chocolate. I decided weddings were a bad idea: no more boyfriends—not that I'd had one, but I planned to—and only white cake.

My only other early encounter with religion was when Mother and Daddy took us to an Easter sunrise service on a hillside outside of Modesto. I thought Easter was all about my new dress and patent leather shoes, plus the See's Candies eggs we would hunt for when we got home. Then I watched the dark sky turn from steely gray to mauve with streaks of orange as the sun came over the hill. Mother held my hand and cried quietly, and I realized beauty could make you cry. Perhaps religion wasn't all bad ideas.

Recalling this years later, I reconsidered whether those kind Dallas clergymen might have something to teach me after all. I retrieved that one-page CCS guide and read it again:

Every woman has four options when faced with a problem pregnancy:

1. Continue the pregnancy, have a baby, and raise a child.
2. Continue the pregnancy and give the baby up for adoption.
3. Abort the pregnancy.
4. Commit suicide.

Those ministers had drafted a revolutionary position: pregnancy should not be synonymous with childbearing. Instead, it presents a woman with choices. The CCS clergymen also recognized the desperation felt by unwillingly pregnant women in midcentury America. Rather than leave it unspoken, they included suicide on their list. It was the only course of action the clergy could not support; the other three options were seen as equally valid moral choices.

I was learning that my religious beliefs, or lack thereof, were beside the point. The patient had to live with her decision, and I would have to live with my role in it. Although I did not believe abortion was a sin, I did see it as an act of conscience—determined by the sense of right and wrong that guides a person's thoughts and actions—for the patient and for me.

The opportunity to develop a new kind of counseling was intriguing to me. It appealed to my independent, creative streak. I knew it would be essential to keep the sessions brief. The feminists had a point: patients did not come for psychotherapy—they came to end a pregnancy. But I already had a sense of the emotionally loaded issues that are closely linked to abortion: feelings about sex and relationships, plans for the future, fears about future fertility, the impact of a stranger (the doctor) probing the vagina and uterus. Abortion was not the straightforward task I had imagined; it is a potential minefield for both patients and those of us providing the care. I needed to create an emotional connection with each patient that would allow these issues to surface quickly without invading their privacy or increasing their anxiety.

I had found a challenging task that would allow me to do good work while distracting me from the dissolution of my marriage. Abortion work had an added bonus for me: given Rob's feelings about abortion, choosing this job virtually ensured that I would get my divorce.

I also brought some hard-won sensitivities to the task. From my own childhood, I knew that parenthood is not only a joy; it is also a solemn responsibility and one that can overwhelm some parents. From my work with marginalized groups, I knew that too many people live without hope because blessings I had taken for granted—a loving family, good education, good health and health care—are not equally available. I also believed that not all pregnancies were "meant to be." This perspective informed my abortion work from the start, particularly my belief that only the pregnant woman is qualified to decide the fate of her pregnancy. What's more, I knew—from my efforts to teach essentially illiterate students in LA and Dallas, which had transformed my love of literature into a deep appreciation for the power of telling one's own story and being heard—that the most important part of my job was to be a good listener.

I was fuzzy, however, on the actual role Dr. Boyd played in the clinic that bore his name but not his presence. I knew only that he lived in New Mexico and visited occasionally. Since I liked the other staff members and the two doctors whom he had trained—both OB-GYN residents at St. Paul's, the Catholic hospital near the clinic—I gave Dr. Boyd no further thought.

In my second week on the job, I finished a counseling session and escorted the patient to the surgery area, where she would meet the doctor who would perform her abortion. As we walked to the surgery room, a bearded man entered the hallway through the back door. He was dressed in bell-bottom jeans, a flowered vest, and round rimless glasses. I assumed he was a friend of the doctor scheduled to do surgery that morning, but the man's appearance rattled my patient.

"Who is that strange man," she asked, "and why is he here?"

So I did what any good feminist would do: I took matters in hand, walking up to the stranger and instructing him to wait for the doctor on the back porch.

He smiled. "Perhaps you don't know who I am." He seemed amused, but I was not.

"Who you are doesn't really matter," I replied. "You're inappropriately dressed for the surgery area, and you're frightening a patient. Please step outside."

He cocked his head, clearly taking my measure, but obeyed.

Later that day, I learned that the hippie I'd thrown out of the clinic was the elusive Dr. Curtis Boyd.

Although this was hardly an ideal introduction, I was still unfazed. I remained confident that I had done the right thing in putting a patient's concerns first. But I had no idea that I had found my calling in this work—and no inkling that I had met the man I would one day choose to wed.

CHAPTER FOUR

An Unexpected Love Story: Creating Our World and Our Workplace

"As life throws you curve balls us women need to stand strong and fight through it all. Sometimes we can't handle everything thrown at us. Be strong and thankful to those supporting you through this. My boyfriend has held my hand the whole way and I have not shown him the thanks and appreciation he deserves. You are not alone. . . . Breathe relax and know we are in it together."

—*Patient journal entry*

Glenna

When I blithely threw Curtis out of his own clinic, I had no idea what he had been through to create the first legal abortion facility in Texas. I knew nothing of the courage or foolhardiness of his actions, nor could I imagine how lonely his journey had been. More to the point, I was in no mood to care. I was separating—yet again, and for the last time—from my husband, Rob. I was short on sympathy for men and lost in a grief that I could not name.

At age twenty-six, I was both a product of my time and not. As a child, I'd renounced fairy-tale weddings and baby carriages. I wanted to be going somewhere, first on my bicycle and roller skates, then with an education, a career, and travel. Love and marriage were not on my personal agenda, and by the time I was sexually active, free love and open marriage were the cultural values of the moment. In photos from the late 1960s and '70s, I look like the consummate flower child with my long blond hair and flawless skin without a trace of makeup. Yet the freewheeling "Love the One You're With," an anthem of my era, was not my song—for reasons I'd yet to examine closely.

It is painful to look back on my teens and early twenties. Those years were still romanticized in my day, so I kept my troubles to myself. I was an imposter, presenting a confident facade to mask the fear and confusion I felt inside. Many of the choices I made were designed to avoid major life decisions.

My first marriage allowed me to delay graduate school and experiment with jobs, long before gap years and work-study programs were accepted practice. I had known before we'd even said our vows that the marriage was a mistake, and imagined that knowledge would somehow protect me from pain when we finally split. It didn't. So the depth of sorrow I felt when I finally left Rob in 1974 caught me by surprise. I was losing my best friend since college and hurting a man I genuinely cared about. I was doing what needed to be done, but it was harder than I'd imagined possible. I felt guilty and lost.

Work was my respite, a place where I could lose myself in helping others and feel safe in the company of women—until Curtis appeared.

My first conversation with Curtis took place the day after I expelled him from the surgery area. I was finishing a patient chart when he peeked around the partition and asked if I had a few minutes to talk. He sat down across the desk and launched into what I would come to know as his standard intake interview: Where had I grown up? What did my parents do? Where had I gone to university? What were my grades?

At the time, I thought he was a typical male establishing his dominant status while also giving me an opportunity to apologize for my error the previous day. I was not going to apologize.

However, when he asked me about my longer-term plans, he had me in a bind. I planned to stay in Dallas only until my divorce was final, but I didn't want to tell my new employer that I was marking time until I could make my getaway—especially since I was committed to the cause and loving the work. I parried the question by talking about my wish to return to graduate school to earn my PhD in psychology. He wasn't fooled. "You didn't answer my question," he said. "What I want to know is how long you plan to stay."

He was sharper than I'd thought.

. . . .

When it came to special attention from men, I was ambivalent at best— and hostile at my worst. Right then, I was at my worst.

From the start, I sensed that Curtis was intrigued by me, perhaps even smitten. He watched me as I went about my work and told me that he'd read the patient thank-you notes collecting in my employee file. "You're exactly what I've been looking for in a counselor," he said. I suspected he was looking for more—saying one thing while meaning another. I couldn't trust him.

He seemed unaware that I was a no-fly zone for men. At the time, he worked mostly in Santa Fe, where his children lived with their mother, and visited the Dallas clinic once a month. On one of those visits, he invited me to dinner.

I thought, *Do you come on to all your new employees?* But I said, "No, thank you."

A week or two later, Curtis invited me to lunch along with other staff who knew and admired him. That lunch was occasioned by a visit from a Texas legislator who supported abortion rights. In 1974, the recently legalized right to abortion had firm, if quiet, support within Texas political circles. Yet sexual harassment in the workplace was not yet recognized as a problem—it was business as usual. As we walked back to the clinic after lunch, the legislator grabbed my left buttock, and I literally growled as I wrenched myself out of his grip.

Later that afternoon I vented my outrage on Curtis, my voice shaking as I recounted what had happened. He simply listened; the sadness on his face spoke for him. He didn't dismiss the event with the platitudes of the time: *I'm sure he didn't mean any offense* or *Come on, that's what men do*. He simply said, "I'm sorry. That must happen too often." His tone was sympathetic, not veiled flattery. Curtis's calm in the face of my upset was reminiscent of my father's quiet way of soothing merely by being with me, and I felt my attitude toward him softening.

I also genuinely appreciated the value Curtis placed on counseling. He told me that the patients he'd seen through the Clergy Consultation Service, where counseling was routine, had seemed at peace with their decision—far less fearful during the abortion procedure than patients who found his office through other channels. Then abortion became legal and the CCS became inactive, so patients were now referred by their own physician, a friend, or a listing in the Yellow Pages. Curtis confessed that his own attempts at group counseling had produced only awkward silence. So, he had stuck to what he did so well—nearly painless surgery combined with silent attention to patients' nonverbal cues—and hired eager, well-intentioned feminists to accompany patients through every step of the abortion process. But those employees were not getting the same results I was. Now Curtis wanted to formalize counseling as an integral part of abortion care.

What's more, working with Curtis in the surgery room was a joy. We communicated easily and usually without words. After meeting privately with the patient, it was my job to escort her to the procedure room and introduce her to the doctor. As she changed into a medical gown, I would set up for the procedure—a task performed by registered nurses (RNs) today—preparing the sterile tray of medical instruments and getting the patient hooked up to an IV line. If a patient tensed when Curtis entered the room, I could nod to him, and he would join me at the head of the exam table to make eye contact and place the palm of his hand on the patient's shoulder. Then he'd walk to the foot of the table and remain standing between her draped legs as I prepared her by saying, "Now you'll feel Dr. Boyd's gentle touch." I spoke with the patient throughout the procedure about anything that interested her, while also functioning as a surgical assistant to the doctor.

Curtis's touch was slow and deliberate. He waited until her body relaxed before he seated himself between the patient's feet, disappearing from her view. Then he worked so quickly that the procedure was often over before the patient realized he'd begun. His interaction with the patient was personalized yet silent—almost ghostlike. His hands and the instruments made no sounds or unnecessary contact with the patient's body. I referred to the whole phenomenon as Dr. Boyd's No-Touch Abortion.

While Curtis was physically gifted in the surgery room, I was more adept at navigating the patient's emotional world—exploring the varied meanings of pregnancy and the impact of her decision to abort in the routine counseling session immediately preceding the abortion. Although I was careful not to suggest that patients needed to justify their decisions or reveal intimate details of their personal life, I was surprised by how much information they volunteered. Then I used my understanding to assist both the patient and the doctor throughout the procedure.

Curtis saw that patients trusted me and that I could transfer that trust to others, including him. He had already started coming to Dallas more frequently, and he always stepped in to work with technically or emotionally challenging patients. Soon those difficult cases became part of my unofficial focus in Dallas as well. Our friendship developed as we worked together in the procedure room more and more often.

We had many conversations in those first months, and although Curtis talked about a comprehensive philosophy of care, he struggled to articulate it. Instead, he told stories from his experience, with a recurrent theme: the importance of treating every patient with respect, even those who were difficult.

One day, Curtis happened to be observing in the surgery area the day a patient sat up on the table, stuck her finger down her throat, and vomited all over me as soon as the procedure was over. The surgeon working that morning had refused to give her additional pain medication because he accurately judged her a drug seeker. Angry, the patient had retaliated against me. I was shocked by her behavior, but I simply went home to shower and change into clean clothes so I could finish my workday. Curtis noticed that as bristly as I could be with him, I was unfailingly tolerant with patients. I clearly held myself to the same professional standard he espoused.

When we had first talked about abortion counseling, I had summarized the essential point of Curtis's stories by expressing my agreement that the most important thing every staff member could do was treat each patient with respect. In turn, our regard could bolster their own self-respect. It was as if I'd put words to his vision, and his vision was grand enough to hold real appeal for me.

"Abortion is ultimately not about the medical procedure," Curtis insisted. "It's about women's place in society and the way women feel about themselves."

When I agreed, he knew I understood. But could I develop a counseling program that would train others to do what I seemed to do naturally?

Curtis was sincere about developing this program together. The seamless ease with which we worked together whenever he was in Dallas showed me that he was a team player who truly wanted a teammate, and we had begun to finish each other's sentences when we spoke. When he asked if I would train other counselors, I said yes. I had no idea what it would lead to.

As soon as I agreed to train counselors, Curtis moved back to Dallas. His move made no sense to me, so I asked what had prompted him to leave Santa Fe, a city I knew he loved. His reply stunned me. "I wanted to court you, of course."

"Courtship" was not in my vocabulary. We had never even had a formal date. But Curtis was disarming and unlike anyone I'd ever known. Still, I treated his declaration as if he were joking. "You must be crazy!" I laughed.

He replied with ease, "Of course. Tell me something I don't know."

. . . .

Long before my divorce, my history with men had been complicated. My parents' marriage had been a full partnership marked by deep understanding of each other and commitment. I had taken their sort of union for granted, and as a young child, I'd been jealous. They snuggled in a way neither of them snuggled with me. I didn't understand that their special cuddle was sexual. I was just mad about being left out.

That was before I was raped.

As a nine-year-old, I had no words for what happened to me, but I knew it was wrong. My father never touched me in that way. I knew my parents saved naked touch for each other, and when I listened at their door, they made happy sounds—murmurs, not snarled orders. What the old man who owned the big house at the corner of our block did to me hurt. When I escaped from him and that eerie house where he had turned off every light, I knew my father was the person to turn to. Going to Mother could make the event a big deal, and I couldn't handle that. My first duty was still to protect her. Daddy would make my world right again, without any fuss.

I ran straight for home, stopping only when I reached the safety of our driveway, where I sorted out my shorts and shirt so nothing looked out of place. I found my father in our garage, putting training wheels on Eddy's bicycle, and I perched gingerly on his work stool to watch. Eventually my heart stopped pounding, and I asked Daddy—in the middle of a late summer afternoon—to teach me to wash dishes.

I know he sensed that something was amiss because as we walked across our big back lawn, he put his hand on my shoulder and said in his quiet, wry tone, "You sure are being a good girl." He was giving me an opening to talk, but I couldn't. I knew he would tell Mother because they talked about everything. Equally important, I needed to forget what had happened. I now had a secret to keep—even from myself.

Daddy drew a sink of warm, soapy water and taught me to do the dishes while we reviewed my multiplication tables. By the time we'd dried the silver and put everything away, the buzzing in my head had stopped. I hoped the sudsy water had somehow washed me clean.

Obviously, coming to terms with my rape would not be so simple, but as a nine-year-old, I couldn't know that. Although I was never raped again, I experienced the garden-variety sexual abuse so many children—boys as well as girls—endure.

The following year, the principal of my elementary school excused me from class each day to be his honorary secretary during the school secretary's lunch hour. I was instructed to sit in his lap and answer his phone. Meanwhile, he fiddled with his zipper—I can still see the white pinstripe on his gray serge slacks. I finally escaped by suggesting to the secretary that I could get his lunch instead and then do the filing she hated. Lap-phone duty fell to a more obedient girl in my class. I felt nauseated, but my scheme worked, and I spent both fifth and sixth grades as the secretary's assistant. I was learning to protect myself from abuse, but I felt guilty—I knew what was going on in the principal's office.

"Special attention" from men continued—from the friends' fathers who stroked my face or hair to strange men who followed me on the street. This was simply a girl's life in the 1950s, and no one talked about it.

So, I kept my fear to myself, but having a boyfriend became essential to my safety plan. In high school, I dated a boy who was older and away at university. Daryl was self-absorbed and arrogant enough to think of me as his property—on call for a date whenever he came home. That arrangement served my purpose. His attitude ensured that I would never really care about him; fed my growing anger toward male entitlement; and most important, made me unavailable. Tucked away on the girlfriend shelf, I felt safe and in control. I was free to form genuine friendships with boys as I chose, something rare for girls of my generation.

When I finished high school, I dumped Daryl. He showed up on my doorstep one Friday evening, expecting me to be available, and I introduced him to a pharmacy student from a nearby university—my date for the night. We walked off and left Daryl standing at the door. Even my mother, who had never liked him, was appalled by my casual cruelty. As for me, my accumulated resentment worked as insulation, protecting me from guilt.

Rob had provided four more years of cover through college, but with him I also experienced friendship and a warm, delightful sexual relationship. Like so many first loves, it had run its course by the end of college. We married anyway. As Rob's wife, I was safe from other men, and I didn't have to chart my own future—something I wasn't ready to do. Clearly, I would follow my husband. I was an imposter, again, and it worked, but at a price: I was using him, and I knew it.

As a young adult, I felt angry and mistrustful with men while continuing to see myself as the innocent victim I had once been. Divorce now forced me to see the harm I was inflicting on others and on myself. I could no longer use men as human shields, but I didn't know another way to feel safe in the world. I was doubly soiled—by the rape and then by my way of coping with it—and doubly vulnerable. I couldn't trust men, but I also no longer trusted myself. I grasped much of this at the time, but it was such painful self-knowledge that it has taken me years and a gifted therapist to gain enough perspective to forgive myself.

Curtis's move to Dallas allowed us to work together almost daily for much of 1974. He courted me with his kindness to patients and his patience with me. I needed that time and those day-to-day interactions to believe that he was one of the truly good men. Fortunately, the love and trust I felt with my father had never wavered. I had genuine friendships, too, with several of my married male professors and their wives. So, I knew good men existed, but I also knew there was no oversupply.

That hard-won knowledge ultimately worked in Curtis's favor.

. . . .

Curtis gave me time, but he never gave up. After a while, I started saying yes to an occasional invitation to dinner. I had never thought of eating together as a form of intimacy, but when I finally met a man who could eat more dessert than I could, I began to sense danger. After one particularly fun and funny meal—Curtis sent the waiter away and insisted on teaching me how to bone a red snapper at a restaurant dinner table—I was worried. I was OK with his romantic interest in me but not with mine in him. I could fall for this man.

Returning to my apartment together that night, I decided that I had to drive him away. Now.

"What do you want from me?" I asked as he sat next to me on the couch.

Curtis was clear. "I want us to live together in a fully committed partnership."

I explained that I was not ready, that I was in fact a bad bet in the commitment department. In what I've come to know as classic Curtis fashion, instead of backing off, he asked for more.

"Actually, I want three things," he said. "I want to grow old with you, I want to become a good father, and I want to have a happy childhood."

I started to laugh, but he was so earnest and vulnerable—as well as absurd—that my laughter turned to tears. I was, yet again, disarmed.

Luck was on his side. Just as my defensive walls were coming down, Curtis's children were scheduled to visit. Knowing what a sucker I am for children, he asked if I would help keep them entertained. They were five, seven, and nine years old, and I quickly understood why Curtis wanted help.

I met them at his apartment complex swimming pool, where Curtis Jr. and Lori, the older two, were trying to drown each other. Curtis did not swim, so I dove in to separate them. By the time I'd wrestled Curtis Jr. away from Lori, we'd formed a physical bond. Lori was spitting up water but breathing, and I was literally in deeper than I'd intended.

Kyle, the youngest, was quiet and watchful—with one notable exception. Later, when we entered Luby's Cafeteria for dinner, he screamed to the room at large, "She's not my mother!"

I laughed and knelt beside him, saying, "We both know I'm not your mother, and I bet no one else cares."

Kyle stopped yelling but remained aloof, and I ached for him. The pain of my own divorce was fresh, but it had been my choice. The children had no choice when their parents had separated three years earlier, and they each showed their pain in different ways. For me, they were a seductive combination of smart and active, inquisitive and troubled.

By the end of the day, they all wanted to snuggle into bed with us for one of Dad's bedtime stories. Curtis's tactic had worked. I fell for his children before I allowed myself to fall in love with him.

Curtis's next bit of good fortune was an opportunity to meet my mother. She was planning a trip to Santa Fe, and I was going to join her for a few days since my father was not coming. Curtis believed you could learn a lot about a woman by knowing her mother, so he was eager to meet mine. When he learned that I was booking a hotel for the trip, he insisted on acting as her host: she would stay in his apartment behind the Santa Fe office while he stayed with old friends. He devoted himself to my mother's agenda, visiting museums, tracking down Native American potters whose work she admired, and exploring Pueblo ruins. They had so many shared interests that my presence seemed nearly incidental.

On our last evening together, when it was just Mother and me, she took my shoulders in her hands, as she had when I was a child in need of scolding. "This is a very decent man, and he loves you," she said. "Don't you dare hurt him the way you always hurt men."

I was devastated. When I told Curtis, expecting his sympathy, he literally bounced up and down, saying, "She likes me! She likes me!" He had won my mother's stamp of approval.

What she'd actually said to me was "You've finally met your match." In her eyes, Curtis was a true fit for me, and equally important, she thought he could handle her headstrong daughter. But Mother had also read my mind and hit my rawest nerve: I was learning to trust Curtis, but I didn't yet trust myself.

Ironically, divorce had taught me that I valued marriage. I wanted an enduring relationship, a pair-bond. I thought of it in that animal way, which stirred a memory: When I was in first grade, a pair of mockingbirds nested in a tree behind our home. I was oblivious to them, far more interested in my new roller skates, until I heard one of the birds crying from the top of their tree. This went on for days, and one afternoon I found my mother watching the bird with tears on her cheeks.

"What's so sad?" I asked.

Mother explained that something had happened to his mate, and he was calling for her. The female bird was dead, and he was heartbroken without her. In hindsight, I believe my mother was crying about the loss of her father—my parents' marriage was strong and intact—but that image and the sound of the mockingbird's cry stayed with me. I was afraid that love could break my heart. The closer I came to loving Curtis, the more afraid I felt. Curtis was ready to risk heartbreak. I was not.

In the face of my resistance, Curtis made a plan. As I would learn, he always has a plan—or several.

My divorce had been final for months, and he knew I was eager to leave Texas, so he started looking at properties in the mountains around Santa Fe. When he invited me to spend a long weekend house hunting in northern New Mexico, I reminded him that I intended to return to California, although I'd made no move in that direction. Instead of arguing the point, he simply asked, "What harm could it do to look at homes in Santa Fe?" We could spend time with his children, whom I adored, and I could use the experience as a house-hunting tutorial. I succumbed.

After two days of looking, though, I said, "None of these are places I would want to live, but I think you—"

I got no further, because Curtis declared his intention: "I'm not interested in anyplace you won't live with me."

Curtis's unwavering belief in his own vision and willingness to risk failure had enabled him to provide abortions before they were legal. Now those same qualities allowed him to overcome my resistance to making a commitment. In my inner turmoil, I had sent enough mixed messages that he believed his determination could prevail. We had even revealed our relationship to the clinic staff, despite my initial misgivings.

From Curtis's perspective, he had invested a year in this courtship—his count began the day he met me. So, he delivered a challenge: "You've been indecisive long enough. If we don't live together, we'll never know what we can create together." His final pitch was so absurd that I laughed when he said it: "I'm really easy to live with."

"No, Curtis, you are not easy," I replied. "But you may be worth it."

To this day, Curtis believes that is the highest compliment I have ever paid him. It's not. But that is how we began the search for what would become our first home together.

· · · ·

I don't think I truly appreciated Curtis's isolation until decades later. He never spoke of his loneliness in the years before we met; he simply does not complain, and I think he was inured to the solitary nature of his life. I knew he was exhausted from the strain of providing illegal abortions for so long, so when he proposed that we move to a scenic mountain village near Santa Fe, I imagined he was already planning a period of retreat. Today, he recalls a very different story.

I had finally agreed to live with him, but our relationship was far from what he dreamed it could be. He wanted me to love him as much as he loved me and imagined that if he spirited me far enough away from my familiar world, he could make his dream come true. It was a strategy straight out of the nursery rhyme "Peter, Peter, Pumpkin Eater." He put his wife in a pumpkin shell, and there he kept her very well. Curtis wanted to take care of me—the primary responsibility of a man in his childhood culture. But I didn't want or need what he'd been raised to offer.

My fiercely independent streak was both confusing and a relief to him. He was determined to find an idyllic place where our relationship could take root and grow. Over the ensuing years I realized that forming our relationship was such a deep need in Curtis that it is the only thing that ever displaced, for a time, his commitment to work. As we dedicated ourselves to building our bond, however, we unwittingly built a partnership that also transformed *his* work into *our* work.

On our search for the best site for the pumpkin shell, Curtis took me and his children to the end of a very long dirt road to a grass-covered meadow surrounded by twenty-five acres of forest. This land was in turn surrounded by national forest and a land grant, so nothing could be built nearby. It had a spectacular view of the Truchas Peaks to the north and the Jemez Mountains to the west. As we wandered the property, with

Curtis reciting the nursery rhyme, the children played hide-and-seek in a thicket of scrub oak trees. Suddenly they emerged from the trees and came running across the meadow, shouting, "We've found your house!"

Hidden among the tangle of oaks were the remains of an adobe farmhouse. The roof was long gone, and years of winter snow and summer rain had melted the mud brick walls to waist height, with portions of window frames still embedded and a rotted wooden door hanging from rusted hinges. Trees had taken root within the walls, but the footprint of what we soon called Hansel and Gretel's cottage remained—complete with the "witch's oven," a New Mexico horno, in what had been a small front yard, and an outhouse in the back.

The children had indeed found our home. Curtis hired a contractor, and we went to work. Within months, we had the Northern New Mexico version of a fairy-tale cottage, so small and remote that none of our friends could believe we were choosing to live there.

We erected a Native American tepee as the children's bedroom for the summer, and Curtis became El Doctor to the older men in the village. Frequently one or another of the men would drop by at dusk, knock at the door, and offer Curtis a swig of whiskey from his hip flask. Curtis would politely take a nip, and then the man, invariably in his seventies or eighties and still working his field each day, would ask for medical advice.

The story was always the same. The man had gone to the new rural health center, where the young doctor on duty had advised him to change his diet and stop drinking whiskey. Did El Doctor, who was older and wiser, agree? Curtis would confirm the man's age and activity level, inquire about his wife and family, and then ask the critical questions, such as "Do you feel like you have a good life?"

"*Sí!*"

"Do you enjoy your meals?"

"*Sí.*"

"Does your whiskey make you feel better or worse?"

"*Mucho más mejor.*"

"Then why would you change what's worked for you all these years?"

"Oh, gracias, El Doctor."

While Curtis was their doctor of choice, I was *la gringa loca*—that "crazy White woman"—because I jogged eight miles each day on the dirt road. These same men waved to me as they worked their land, and we shouted greetings to each other, but I was clearly nuts. Even so, after every snowfall, one or more of the men would come by on a snowmobile to be sure *los norteamericanos* were safe.

I missed working with patients and staff, but falling in love so soon— on the heels of my divorce—required my full attention. I had learned the hard way that marriage is serious business. If I wanted this relationship to work—and I did—then I needed to devote myself to it. Together we hiked for days in the wilderness, and Curtis taught me to garden. The joy of dirt under my fingernails after planting a row of lettuce sprouts was as delicious as the young lettuce I later picked. Weeding that garden may have been my first experience of a truly meditative state. It was an idyllic period. We each healed our wounds and formed the pair-bond that endures to this day.

We married in the meadow at dawn in the fall of 1977, with Lori as maid of honor and Curtis Jr. as best man. Kyle held our rings—dropping them only twice—as our dog, Miguel, stood watch. My mother read a favorite poem from my childhood, "The Owl and the Pussy-Cat." Friends from Texas and New Mexico camped in the meadow, and we invited the whole village to dance to a traditional Hispanic fiddler.

Curtis, the farm boy, had handled me the way a wise horse trainer works with a skittish horse—he gentled me, but he never tried to break my spirit. Much later, I asked him why he put up with my indecision and outright rejections. His answer captured how alone he'd felt. He had been physically attracted to me immediately, but a deeper feeling told him we could have something special if I would allow it to develop. Only years later did he realize why he refused to abandon his quest. "Our conversations," he said, "were unlike any I'd had in my life."

Curtis had grown up in a world where he found the conversations inane and usually slipped away to be alone. By contrast, I engaged my heart and mind when we talked, as I'd learned to do with my parents.

Curtis and I were able to contend with each other, to differ vigorously and learn from each other. We made each other better—not only better informed but also better people.

Indeed, our conversations, whether spirited or more reflective, were special. I love quirky, creative minds, and Curtis has one. Yet as I learned, no one had ever listened to Curtis with the wish to understand his unique point of view. I had always thought of finding one's voice and being heard as a feminist issue, but it was a central issue in Curtis's life too. He found his voice in our conversations—and my belief in the power of listening grew deeper.

I knew our relationship was special, and I wanted it to last. We are both far too intense, not to mention stubborn, to be easy, but we find each other worth the effort required to stay in love. At moments we imagined growing old together in that cottage, needing little more than each other's constant company, the children with us weekly, and occasional visits from family and friends. Of course, it didn't work out that way.

. . . .

In the year following our wedding, so many bad things happened in our personal and professional lives that we can hardly remember them all now. Accidents, injuries, life-threatening surgeries, and deaths befell our family. The religious right, personified by the Moral Majority, decided that opposition to abortion would be their source of political power. The years immediately following legalization had led to a proliferation of abortion clinics in Dallas, some ethical and some not, and all competing for patients.

In 1978, Curtis and I agreed that we needed to return to Dallas. The small Santa Fe clinic was in Reggie's capable hands, with an idealistic young doctor Curtis and I had recruited from the Indian Health Service. The Santa Fe clinic would be fine; the Fairmount Center in Dallas needed our leadership if it was to become the model of professional abortion care we envisioned. We had another reason for moving to Dallas. Curtis was asked to serve on the founding board of directors of the first national professional organization of abortion providers: the National Abortion Federation (NAF). It was crucial that we be in a major US city, especially one with a prestigious medical school and a good airport. The opportunity to shape the future of the field he had worked so hard to legitimize was too important for him to pass up. Eventually Curtis left the board—he had no patience for bureaucracy and little talent in navigating it—and I was recruited in his place. We were once again fully engaged at a local, regional, and now national level in the provision of abortion services. Our social cause had become both a political issue and a business, and we wanted our values to set the standard of care for abortion services. Our retreat was over.

But knowing what we needed to do did not make it easy. We planned to share time between our clinic in Dallas and our home in New Mexico. Curtis would schedule our weekly life with the precision he scheduled staff and patients. However, the travel proved exhausting, and what I described as "weekly culture shock" further drained us. Within months, we left our New Mexico cottage with a caretaker and moved into a residential hotel across the street from the Dallas clinic. It was wrenching to leave our life in the mountains, but our most important work was yet to come.

Our three-year respite had given us the renewed energy for this next phase of our life together. We had learned how to create our own world, and now we approached the workplace in the same way—as a world that could embody our shared values and creative powers. The Fairmount Center became our next labor of love.

While Curtis focused on the development of second-trimester abortion techniques, I concentrated on training both counselors and administrators to represent our values. Although counseling and administration are usually seen as separate skill sets, the best counselors—like administrators—appreciate efficiency, find support in chain of command, and enjoy being part of a good team. Similarly, the most effective administrators care about quality of life of all employees, seeking their opinions and taking pride in (not credit for) work done well by others. At their core, good counseling and administration are both built on the capacity to care about others and place trust in them.

This understanding informed the counseling model I developed, which invites each woman to tell her story in her own voice and then trusts her to make the best decision. That model would set the tone for every aspect of our work. We trust the pregnant woman to make the best decision. In the privacy of the counseling room, we do not sit in judgment; we bear witness.

Most couples are probably not well suited to working together, but when they are, they can create something special. The love and trust inherent in the pair-bond spill over into the workplace, and seeing the other person's abilities in action reinforces the mutual respect between them. For Curtis and me, our commitment to each other extended to a commitment to support our staff through the inevitable hard times in life, both personal and professional. We both have needed to grow emotionally, and we support, even require, such growth in our staff. Owning our mistakes and recognizing our vulnerabilities is valued, not punished. We want everyone to succeed but never at the expense of another. That's what makes a healthy team—whether a marital couple or a whole work group.

We practiced these values daily, in the good manners of *please* and *thank you*, in moments away from patients to cry or laugh or scream, in tag-teaming to manage unpleasant interactions, and in monthly staff meetings in which we blended the learning-from-case-review of medical training with the self-examination of group therapy. This approach seems simple, even self-evident, but it is not common practice in medicine or business.

Several years ago, a colleague in our Albuquerque office confessed something that was said after one of our staff parties, when the employees had lingered at the restaurant after Curtis and I exited early. (Parties are more fun when the bosses aren't around!) In a sentimental moment, one counselor reversed what she'd meant to say, and although I've yet to make the T-shirt, her slip of the tongue captured our ethos. I still remember her words:

"This family feels a lot like a clinic."

Part II

Our Work

CHAPTER FIVE

Out of the Dark: New Techniques and Technologies

"Thank you for giving me a choice as well as a voice. I'm 17 and was in late term [of my pregnancy]. Before I found this place I was lost, alone, and felt like my only option left was suicide. You wonderful women give me a second chance at life. You saved me from myself and for that I am eternally grateful. You are angels on earth. Thank you."
—*Patient journal entry*

Curtis

As I walked out of a medical meeting in 1978, I felt a hand on my elbow. It was Dr. Mildred Hanson, and she spoke with urgency in her voice. "Curtis, could we talk in private?" she asked. "Now."

When abortions became legal in 1973, Millie was one of the first doctors to provide them. Her compassion for patients was as legendary as her stylish suits and high-heeled shoes. She had introduced herself to me the following year at another medical meeting, explaining that she had wanted to provide abortions before they were legal, but as a divorced mother with four young children to raise, she had felt unable to take the risk. Legalization had allowed her to willingly take on the role of medical director for Planned Parenthood of Minnesota, as well as North Dakota and South Dakota, while maintaining her successful private OB-GYN practice.

I had long been impressed by Millie's commitment, not to mention her energy, and grateful for her forthright support of my work before *Roe v. Wade*. Since our first meeting, we had counted each other as friends. Now, as we sat in a hotel lounge at one of the early meetings of the newly formed National Abortion Federation, her eyes brimmed with tears.

The urgent story Millie wished to share involved a young woman who had traveled to Minneapolis seeking an abortion. The pregnancy had been beyond Millie's first trimester limit, and she had reluctantly sent the would-be patient away. That young woman had returned to her hotel room and jumped from the window to her death. Millie learned of the suicide from the front page of the *Minneapolis Tribune*. Months had passed, yet Millie still felt responsible for the woman's tragic suicide. She had resolved to learn to do abortions in the second trimester.

"Would you help me?" she asked.

Millie's vulnerability caught me by surprise and left me speechless. I think Millie turned to me because after abortion was legalized, I had been open about my previous illegal work, and now I was openly working to develop safe techniques for abortion later in pregnancy. My reputation for honesty in such sensitive matters led her to trust me—to trust that I would understand her heartache and her need to do more for desperate patients. She assumed, correctly, that those were my motives too.

In the late 1970s, the second trimester of pregnancy was new territory for office- and clinic-based medical practice. As I silently counted my blessings—to my knowledge, I had not lost a patient to suicide—I assured Millie that I would share everything I learned with her.

Working alone and in secret for so many years had been lonely. The risks, both to patients and to me, had weighed me down, but I had enjoyed the challenge of learning by doing. Being my own teacher had suited me, and I was still learning by doing. With the creation of NAF in 1977, however, I was no longer alone, and neither was Millie. We may have lacked the guidance of more experienced teachers—there were none—but now we had each other.

We were no longer operating in the dark.

NAF was founded shortly after *Roe v. Wade*, when providers from around the country could finally gather to share their experiences, problems, insights, and techniques. Conscientious abortion providers had a shared mission, and together we established the standard of care for first-trimester abortion. In contrast to the pre-*Roe* years, women could go to any clinic in the country and—as long as it was an NAF member—be sure that it would meet our standards of safety.

I had felt honored when I was recruited to be a member of NAF's founding board of directors. In this organization, my prelegal work was clearly not a mark against me. Instead, I was recognized as the closest thing to an expert in an emerging and legitimate field of medicine. The vacuum aspiration technique that I had helped pioneer in the United States had transformed first-trimester abortion into a quick and simple procedure that public health officers at the Centers for Disease Control described as safer than a tooth extraction.[12]

Now that I no longer lived in constant fear, relief mingled with my sense of responsibility to advance the field. When Glenna and I returned to Dallas in 1978, we had a shared mission: to bring the respect we provided to women seeking first-trimester abortions to our care for women further in pregnancy.

· · · ·

Glenna had magically appeared at the Fairmount Center and changed my understanding of counseling. More important to me personally, of course, she had changed my life. During our years of retreat in the mountains, we'd had many long conversations about the moral questions surrounding abortion: *When does life begin? How far in the pregnancy could we perform abortions? How far should we? Who should decide?*

Throughout that period of much-needed respite, we had not been doing the work every day, yet abortion in all its complexity never lost its hold on our hearts and minds. On the contrary, we had the luxury of time for deep reflection on its meaning—for each of us and for society. I wanted to develop second-trimester surgical techniques that would be safe in the clinic, while Glenna wanted to train our entire staff—from receptionists on the phone and at the front desk to nurses in the recovery room—to provide care that reflected a counselor's sensitivity to the full range of patients' feelings.

Since medical school, I had believed that an in-hospital abortion procedure placed an unnecessary physical and emotional burden on patients. All too often, in a setting devoted to the delivery of healthy babies to delighted parents, the distress of these women was ignored. Although I had enjoyed my obstetrical rotations and loved delivering babies in my family practice, the indifference—often bordering on hostility—displayed by many hospital staff toward patients who needed to end their pregnancies had always disturbed me, and there was no indication that the legalization of abortion five years earlier had changed that. In fact, abortion at any gestation remained largely unavailable in US hospitals. If we could provide those later abortions in the clinic, where staff were preselected for their support of abortion rights, we could make an important contribution to women's reproductive health care.

However, second-trimester procedures presented special challenges, as I had discovered in my illegal days. We had no one-size-fits-most standard of care, and for good reasons. Each advancing week of gestation presents new technical challenges for the operator and medical risks for the patient. Remembering my patient Lisa's hysterectomy before abortion was legal, I had hard-earned respect for both types of obstacles. As a responsible physician, I simply did not know how far into this uncharted territory I could safely venture.

The first challenge was dilating the cervix widely enough to allow for safe removal of the larger pregnancy without damaging the cervix in the process. This was of particular concern in the early years because bleeding from cervical tears had been a problem with illegal abortion—as with the unfortunate woman whose abortion I had reported during my internship. None of us in the legal abortion community wanted to perpetuate that problem. And we did not yet have sufficient evidence from legal abortion to put that concern behind us. Scrupulous surveillance of legal abortion by the CDC would eventually eliminate that worry, but we were not there yet. For the patients' well-being and our own, we had to proceed with caution.

Although my dilation technique was gradual and gentle, I needed to stretch the natural opening in the cervix two to three times the diameter required for earlier procedures, so I was always mindful. Once the cervix was dilated, I employed the suction technique that is now standard in early abortion with a larger cannula and then added forceps, plus the curette to assure that no pregnancy tissue was left behind. By combining the widely accepted vacuum aspiration of early abortion with a far more demanding version of the D&C I had mastered in my medical training, we could keep these patients out of the hospital and safely end later pregnancies in our emotionally supportive clinic environment.

Since patient safety was paramount, I wanted a clear idea of what I was getting into. So, in 1978, we became one of the first abortion clinics in the nation to acquire an ultrasound machine. Ultrasound imaging provided a "picture" of the patient's uterus so we could measure the size of the pregnancy growing within. Much like early computers, however, the machine was a behemoth—not only big but also expensive compared with what we use today. Glenna worried about increasing prices, but I knew it would improve safety, and she trusted me not to pass the cost through to our patients.

The salesman trained Glenna to use the machine with ease, and Glenna trained our nurse, Daniece, who became our chief ultrasound technician. Daniece was a petite powerhouse accustomed to getting what she wanted with her wits and her southern drawl. She was also unfailingly compassionate to those in need. However, this new role placed Daniece in the difficult position of turning patients away when their pregnancies were beyond our limit—a particularly heartbreaking task when the pregnancy was only days past our declared limit.

The scenario became worse still when the woman broke down in tears, begging Daniece to reconsider and let her have the abortion, no matter the risk. Daniece would then ask Glenna to verify the ultrasound measurements, and in many cases, they came to me together—in basketball it's called "double teaming." Would I consider performing an abortion for a patient who was three or four days, maybe a week, past our stated limit? They both had confidence in my ability to do the procedure—sometimes more confidence than I felt—or they would not ask. How could I say no when we all thought I could do the procedure safely? In this highly personal way, I gradually extended my gestational limit, constantly refining my technique. As the clinic began expanding our limit, word got out. Women in their eighteenth, twentieth, even twenty-second weeks of pregnancy came to our doors. Now that abortion was legal and we had excellent hospital backup care, I was determined to develop the technical skills to responsibly say yes to these women.

As I pushed the gestational boundary beyond what I had been willing to risk before legalization, my primary concern was preventing damage to the patient's cervix or uterus. While first-trimester procedures are usually quick and simple, abortions later in pregnancy take longer and have an increased risk of complications. Since some complications can impair future childbearing, I wanted to avoid them.

While managing second-trimester patients' pain was another important piece of the puzzle we would have to fit in place, at the time my primary focus was on *safe* surgical techniques. I needed to keep the patient relatively comfortable while I dilated the cervix more widely and emptied the larger uterus with its increased blood supply. I worked on a more effective placement of the local anesthetic, injecting numbing medication into both the cervix and the lower portion of the uterus, in order to block pain fibers in a larger area than the standard cervical block as I'd been taught. This took a little more time but provided better pain control.

With Glenna as the counselor and a skilled RN working together to reassure the patient—and me—we progressed, week by week, further into the second trimester. By the end of the year, I was saying yes to patients who were twenty-four weeks pregnant. My personal motto—*Say yes if you can and no only if you must*—became our clinic motto.

The great truth of pain is that the shorter it lasts, the better we tolerate it. Pain signals danger, and that signal is essential to survival in all animals, including humans. To endure it, we have to override our instinctive response: to recoil. The prolonged procedure taxed the patient's natural instinct and thus our ability to manage her pain effectively. Glenna had learned that most patients did not want to dwell on possible complications, but as the procedure dragged on and they felt more pain, they feared something was wrong. Their worry then intensified their pain—the proverbial vicious circle.

Medicine has long recognized the relationship between anxiety and perceived pain, often using that link to dismiss patient complaints: *It's all in your head.* The usefulness of the link between relaxation and pain tolerance, however, was not given much attention before the 1950s. My own excellent medical training from 1959 to 1964 had treated pain as a purely physical matter to be either anesthetized or endured with stoic dignity. In the absence of knowledge, we relied on intuition—and when I speak of intuition, I am really talking about Glenna.

Glenna knew how to project calm in a surgery room. Her body language was relaxed, her voice soothing. As I worked, I would overhear her talking with patients about the details of their daily lives, their dreams for the future, a favorite place to walk or watch the sunset—anything the patient found peaceful. This was unexpectedly reassuring to me as well.

When the patient felt pain, Glenna responded sympathetically but without alarm. She asked patients to describe the sensation, to locate it in their body: Was it on the left or right? Was it hot or cold? Sharp or dull? She also offered explanations of those sensations to let the patient know that nothing was going wrong: "Those heavier cramps are your uterus quickly shrinking now that it's empty," Glenna would say. "That is a healthy sign and can mean less bleeding after we're finished. Let me know as the cramps begin to ease." Her ability to voice what I cared about but would not put into words allowed both me and the patient to successfully see the procedure through.

I had taught Glenna to ask patients if they wanted me to stop until uncomfortable sensations had passed. This had long been my practice, and I remember a patient for whom I'd stopped mid-procedure. As I prepared to resume, I said, "I'll be touching you again, and you may feel some discomfort."

"It's not discomfort, damn it," the patient snapped. "It's pain!"

Point taken.

Glenna's willingness to take each patient's experience seriously—and to use the word "pain" when the patient did—ran counter to my medical school training. It also worked wonders. I was frankly startled when, after abortion was legal, patients freely expressed their pain. Without Glenna's natural patience and compassion, I might have been stymied by this. In my years of prelegal abortion, I had not recognized that my patients were being so stoic.

Along with Glenna, patients were retraining me and reinforcing my commitment to respect their reality and give them as much control of their abortion experience as medical safety would allow. Several of our counselors were also good bedside coaches and had success with their own intuitive ways of comforting patients. But you can't teach intuition. We needed teachable skills, and that would become our next quest.

· · · ·

I was gratified to have mastered techniques to safely end pregnancies through twenty-four weeks in the clinic. In 1979, I was invited to present my work on the D&E as part of a panel at the University of North Carolina at Chapel Hill School of Medicine. Glenna created a slide presentation by photographing each step of the procedure using a camera with a macro lens.

Glenna got signed consent from each patient she photographed, and we offered to preview that portion of my lecture for their approval. Everyone she asked willingly gave permission and wanted to see the slideshow. When Glenna explained that the close-up photos of their cervix would in no way identify them, she imagined that they would be relieved to remain anonymous. Instead, they were disappointed. The eagerness of these women to go proudly public as abortion patients was a stunning contrast to the secrecy and shame of patients prior to legalization.

The photos captured my innovative approach to cervical dilation in detail—illustrating my use of patience and finesse instead of force. When I showed those slides as I spoke in North Carolina, the doctors on the panel and in the audience were attentive. The photos made the process real, but few could imagine doing what they saw, so I invited them to visit our clinic. Several medical school professors I admired came as their busy schedules allowed, including Dr. Phillip Stubblefield, then at Harvard, and Dr. Philip Darney from University of California San Francisco (UCSF). Both have had distinguished academic careers and made significant contributions of their own to abortion education and quality of care.

Then a private practitioner from Kansas asked to visit. Eventually, that doctor would perform abortions later in pregnancy than I had— and ultimately change our practice in ways none of us could foresee— but at the time, Dr. George Tiller was still learning.

George came to the Dallas clinic in the early 1980s, some years after we met him at an NAF meeting. He had injured his back right before the trip and was in excruciating pain, but he was so committed to expanding his gestational limit that he came anyway. I will always remember George sitting on the hard linoleum floor behind me, propped on one elbow so he could get the best view without bending over. Even in pain, he was the consummate gentleman. After observing the day's procedures, George just shook his head and laughed. "That may work for you, Curtis, but I don't have your hands."

George joked that my nerve endings extended to the tips of my instruments. That extra sensitivity had been a survival skill before 1973, and I value it to this day. Even with the ultrasound machine available, we used it only to verify gestation—not during surgeries as is the norm today. I didn't need to see when I could feel my way through the procedure, and in fact I often worked with my eyes closed. We had a running joke in the clinic that in my old age a nurse could wheel me into the surgery room and I'd continue to work even if I were blind. Although that was never part of my career plan—all notorious medical "humor" aside—my eventual retirement would depend on sharing our experience and know-how with other care providers. At that time, however, retirement was not on my mind. I wanted to teach others to do what I was doing so that second-trimester abortions by D&E would be more widely available to patients in need.

I had always believed George was a good doctor—he'd sat beside me in the front row of every medical meeting lecture we attended together—but this exchange deepened my respect for him. George was not only an earnest student; he also had humility, one of the greatest virtues in the religion of my childhood and essential to the best practice of medicine. Thus, it came as no surprise that George had been raised in a deeply religious community, and his faith would strengthen and sustain him in the hard times to come. As he was learning to perform abortions in the second trimester, his realistic self-assessment combined with his determination enabled him to develop surgical techniques that worked for him. With years of experience, his technique would later allow him to perform abortions into the third trimester.

George's reaction to my surgical technique could have alerted me to the reality: teaching others might not be as easy as I'd hoped.

I knew that I was good with my hands. In medical school I had chosen to work on a burn unit, performing skin grafts freehand as we had no computers to aid the process. It was a dreaded placement among med students because burn patients were in nearly intolerable pain, but I had loved the concentration and precision of my task. On surgical rotations, I noticed that where I relied on technique and finesse, others immediately applied strength and force during a surgical procedure—which could quickly get them, and the patient, into trouble. It dawned on me that during my childhood on the farm, ministering to sick or injured animals and delivering calves as a matter of course, I had acquired a special tactile sensibility that was particularly useful as I taught myself to perform D&Es.

The D&E techniques seem self-evident now, but they were not so in the developmental phase. Looking back, I find the patience and persistence required to manually dilate the cervix daunting, and that was the reaction of most of the doctors who observed me. Successfully teaching would require more than personal determination.

. . . .

The next time I saw Millie, we had our usual warm exchange, but she was not in tears—quite the opposite. She was excited by a new possibility and hoped this time she could help me. She asked a question that would soon change the future of abortion care in the second trimester: "Have you heard of laminaria?"

Laminaria is a type of Japanese seaweed used in everything from cooking to traditional medicines. When dried and compressed, laminaria "tents" look like cigarettes of various widths with strings attached at one end. I knew that laminaria had been used to induce labor since the mid-1800s and that a few physicians were using it in early-abortion procedures. The physician would insert the sterile tent into the patient's cervix, where, over a period of several hours, it would absorb moisture from the woman's body. As the tent expanded, the cervix would soften and open. Laminaria might even induce labor and a miscarriage without surgical intervention—the way the strips of slippery elm my grandmother used could "bring on" a period for women back home in East Texas. Inducing a miscarriage was not my goal. I simply wanted a more teachable technique for the D&E. With so much experience using small mechanical dilators in my training, I'd never seen the benefit of using laminaria. But the greater dilation required for abortions later in pregnancy was a different story.

Millie was intrigued, and so was I. She was planning a trip to Japan to buy laminaria and asked if I would like her to bring me samples. I replied with a grateful "Yes!" And thanks to Millie, a new era in second-trimester abortion began.

Dilation with laminaria was slower than manual dilation, which is why I hadn't considered using it for early procedures. It takes time for the laminaria to expand to the point where the cervix dilates enough for safe extraction: hours in the first trimester, and one or two days in the second trimester. We monitored patients in the clinic during the day, changing laminaria as they progressed, and patients had to arrange to spend the night nearby so we could meet them at the clinic if they went into labor in the night. Although this was time consuming for patients and staff, inserting a laminaria tent was safer and less intimidating for most learners, making it easier for me to teach other doctors.

Like most solutions, however, this created new problems: how many tents to insert, in what combination of sizes, how long to allow them to expand, and so forth. When silicone-based osmotic dilators came on the market several years later, in 1982, they expanded more quickly than the compressed seaweed. This altered the calculus but not the concept, and abortion providers still use both laminaria and silicone dilators today.

Osmotic dilators were a game changer, but they weren't magic. While waiting for their cervix to dilate, patients were uncomfortable at best. Plus, the dilators might fail to expand or—in the worst cases—get stuck and become very difficult to remove manually. Such setbacks were rare, but for everyone's sake, I wanted to avoid them. We needed something more to help the cervix soften and relax, creating the optimum outcomes for both patients and clinical staff.

Years would pass before the arrival of a medication that could do the job.

When misoprostol entered the market in 1988 as a treatment for stomach ulcers, its use was specifically contraindicated in pregnant women because it can cause miscarriages. It was exactly what we needed.

My first strategy was to insert the misoprostol tablet into the vagina the night before surgery so that the misoprostol would work as the patient slept. This seemed like the most logical plan, and it worked. Frequently, in fact, it worked too well.

It is common knowledge that women sometimes deliver babies in awkward, if not dangerous, places, and that can happen with abortion as well. Our on-call staff would receive a desperate call in the middle of the night from a patient in labor. The on-call nurse and counselor would rush to the office to meet me. We would turn off alarms, flip on lights, draw up medications, and set up the instrument tray. The patient would arrive, and in minutes we could complete the procedure. Medically speaking, this was simple, but it was emotionally stressful for both the patient and our staff.

Worse, sometimes the patient couldn't get to the office in time. She might pass the pregnancy at home, in a motel room, or in the car en route to the clinic. Our staff handled these events with kindness and grace, providing the best care possible under sometimes chaotic circumstances. However, this was not how we wanted things to go.

One teenage patient agreed to spend the night within thirty miles of the clinic, but to save money, she ended up going to her mother's home in a small town west of Fort Worth—some sixty miles from Dallas. Her mother called in the night and drove her daughter to the clinic *after* she expelled the pregnancy at home. I completed the procedure in the clinic while Glenna drove several hours round-trip to retrieve the fetus in accord with public health standards.

For us, it was all in a day's work. However, most of our patients had enough trauma in their lives. So I experimented with doses and timing until I came to a solution: Rather than give the misoprostol dose when we inserted the dilators, intending it to work overnight, we gave it the following morning and asked the patient to remain in our clinic for monitoring. Then, when her cervix was ready, we would perform the extraction. No more middle-of-the-night surprises—problem solved.

There is an expression in obstetrics: *The cervix is queen!* In abortion care we, too, wisely obey the "queen." As we listened to the needs of the patient and her body, our cervical dilation process evolved with experience and technology.

So did our approach to pain management. Glenna continued to work on effective counseling during the procedure and what would later be labeled "nonpharmacological" pain management. Meanwhile, I turned to the pharmacy.

We wanted the safest, most effective drugs for use in an outpatient clinic so our patients could be as comfortable as possible and still recover quickly. I hired an anesthesiologist as a consultant, and he recommended combining a fast-acting sedative (versed) with a pain blocker (fentanyl). By combining the two medications, we could use a smaller dose of each, thus increasing safety; this also created a "potentiating" effect, with each drug making the other more effective. Additionally, by administering the medications in a very slow intravenous push, our trained medical staff could watch the effect on each patient and give only as much as needed. Once again, by tailoring our intervention to each patient's need, we improved outcomes for all patients.

Our goal in developing the D&E as a safe in-office procedure for second-trimester abortion had been to spare patients the potential trauma of labor and delivery on a hospital ward devoted to bringing healthy babies into the world. Patients at any stage of pregnancy may believe they will look back on their need for an abortion with regret for what might have been—if only their pregnancy had been healthy, or their own life or relationship or health had been different. But we wanted patients to feel good about themselves and find comfort in the care they received from us. We wanted all of our patients, regardless of their reasons for needing an abortion or their gestation, to be treated with respect—not as failed women, or as women fallen from the grace of God or that of their community—as they navigated an important life decision.

It had taken a full decade longer than I'd expected, but with the advent of osmotic dilators and misoprostol, we finally achieved the goal Millie and I had envisioned: developing a teachable second-trimester surgical technique. By the end of the 1980s, however, the new generation of doctors committed to abortion care that we had expected had not materialized.

. . . .

I had taught myself, the doctors who worked for us, and a few doctors with already established abortion services. But the majority of providers were the early adopters, and by 1990, many of us were old White men going bald or gray. This general absence of younger doctors to carry on the work was worrisome.

Throughout my training, medicine had been a fraternity—a male do-main. Women medical school graduates would not achieve near parity with men until 2007 or 2008, and today nearly equal numbers of men and women graduate from medical school. By contrast, there were only three women graduates in my med school class of 1965.

As I was developing the D&E as a teachable skill set in the late 1980s, women physicians were slowly entering the workforce: 25 percent of med school graduates in 1980 were female, and by 1990 that figure had grown to 33 percent.[13] But the women physicians we had always hoped for were not choosing to perform abortions in sufficient numbers to achieve the workforce needed for the future.

The potential workforce shortage was so concerning that the major pro-choice organizations and several prestigious foundations spon-sored a retreat for leaders in the field to address "the graying of abor-tion" in America.

For this symposium, Glenna and I were selected to represent in-dependent abortion providers, and we helped identify the barriers to younger doctors entering the field. Foremost among our concerns were the lack of abortion care training in medical schools and residency pro-grams, and the stigma perpetuated by that exclusion from mainstream medical training.

UCSF's Dr. Philip Darney was one of the other participants in that 1990 symposium. He also believed that medical education had to in-clude abortion as a necessary skill in OB-GYN training. Dr. Uta Landy, a psychologist with a deep understanding of providing abortion services from her early work in Austria and from her years as the executive di-rector of NAF, developed a plan and sought funding for what would be-come the Ryan Residency Training Program and the Ryan Fellowship in Family Planning. Starting with the Women's Options Center train-ing program at UCSF as the pilot, the Ryan Program changed medical training in the OB-GYN departments of more than one hundred med-ical schools. A similar, smaller program in family medicine residencies also emerged.

This work within existing medical training systems was key to legit-imizing abortion as essential to women's health care across the United States and around the world.[14] Women who needed to end their preg-nancies were getting safer care than was possible before 1973—and we believed that ensuring the education of future providers meant that trend could continue indefinitely. Meanwhile, the ongoing work of the CDC's Abortion Surveillance Division, tasked with monitoring the health problems associated with legal abortion, unintentionally docu-mented the overwhelming safety of legal abortion following *Roe v. Wade*.

The role of the CDC in the public health of the nation and the world has expanded far beyond its original charge. Various CDC branches have monitored and evaluated responses to public health issues, from seasonal flu vaccines to radioactive contamination after Three Mile Is-land. Most Americans alive today are familiar with the agency due to its highly visible role in the AIDS epidemic of the 1980s and the Covid-19 pandemic of the early 2020s. But the Division of Reproductive Health had also studied risks to women's health surrounding the birth con-trol pill, the IUD (intrauterine device), and estrogen replacement ever since the 1960s. After the legalization of abortion in 1973, the CDC had carefully followed my work and that of other abortion providers.

The National Public Health officers in charge of that division at the time, Dr. David Grimes and Dr. Willard Cates, worked without religious or political agendas. They followed the facts and in doing so made a huge contribution to women's health in the United States.

We have reported all abortions performed at our clinics since 1973 with full details of all medical complications. The data from many abor-tion facilities like ours, combined with careful analysis by CDC officials, allowed providers (and the public) to evaluate the safety and effective-ness of new products and innovations. Legal abortion in the United States had created a market for improved medical devices, and the CDC's careful analysis accelerated the development and adoption of brand-new technologies and techniques that benefited countless patients. The agency's review of surgical outcomes in US clinics quickly established that abortion by vacuum aspiration was superior to the D&C and that the D&E was superior to the hospital-based induction of labor for management of abortion in the second trimester. The Abortion Surveillance System's monitoring of abortion procedures continues to this day.

. . . .

Through those years of constant change, naturally I attended to the medical pieces of the puzzle, eager to make abortions safe and doable, with an eye on ensuring the future of abortion care. We now had the cutting-edge technology and surgical techniques to perform abortions through the second trimester. Together, we could savor the D&E as mission accomplished and face future challenges as a team, taking pride in our work.

My focus, as always, was on the critical medical question: *Is this procedure safe?* But this bypassed the deeper philosophical questions: *Is it "right"?* and *Am I comfortable doing it?*

I was slow to appreciate how much I was asking of our staff. Those who had been with us since we opened after *Roe* had been accustomed to abortions up to fourteen weeks performed by all of our doctors, and up to seventeen weeks when I was available. They worked comfortably within those limits; this was their normal. As I increased my skills through determination and the aid of new technology, we slowly but steadily extended our gestational limit—from seventeen weeks to twenty-four weeks. Each change in our gestational limit required new protocols and disrupted the status quo—creating uncertainty and fear among our staff.

As usual, I left such matters to Glenna. I knew that she considered these questions seriously and was attending to the evolving needs of both patients and staff. Looking forward, she had a problem to solve that was entirely different from mine: how to help counselors and medical staff adjust to our changing protocols so the procedures would be emotionally and psychologically manageable—not just for patients but for us too.

CHAPTER SIX

Precious, Glowing Things: Attending to Our Feelings

"There are not enough words to describe the things that I feel at this moment. To make the right decision is yet to be clear to me. A part of me feels like a monster, another part of me feels like this was the best decision I could have made. Life has such an amazing and powerful way of waking you up inside. I believe that someday it will all make sense. This will stay with me forever. I will never forget. But I know, I know in my heart that I will be okay. Please lord forgive me, I hope that one day I can forgive myself."
—Patient journal entry

Glenna

When I began this work in 1974, I had a prejudice against abortions later in pregnancy. How could a woman wait so long? Fear of unintended pregnancy had been ever present since my first sexual intercourse.

In 1965, when I was a freshman in college, the thrill of orgasm with my boyfriend outweighed my fear—and we did use a condom—but from that first time on, I tracked my menstrual periods on the calendar and sighed with relief when I bled. The calendar method worked for me until my favorite college roommate confided in me that she had been date-raped after her high school prom. In her desperation to keep this shameful secret from her prominent, devoutly Catholic family, she'd flown to Mexico City for an abortion—under the pretext of a summer holiday before she started college. Her whole abortion experience was traumatic, beginning with the rape and continuing through months of post-abortion bleeding, until the kindly doctor at our student health center arranged for her to get a D&C and a blood transfusion for acute anemia. I can still see her sitting up in bed in the campus clinic, pale but finally recovering.

I didn't want that.

So I made an appointment with my mother's gynecologist during summer vacation. I wanted birth control pills, which had just become legal across America in the landmark Supreme Court case *Griswold v. Connecticut*—for married couples, anyway.

As Mother's doctor performed my first pelvic exam, he said, "So are you married, getting married, or just playing married?" He made no eye contact, and I heard the smirk in his voice.

Naked from the waist down, covered with a small white sheet, with his right hand in my vagina as his left hand poked hard against my belly, I was furious.

As soon as his hand was out of me, I yanked my feet from the stirrups, sat up to face him, and said, "None of the above, and none of your business. Are you going to write the prescription or not?"

The doctor simply turned and walked from the room, slamming the door behind him. I imagined him calling my mother—they were friends. What would she think? I frankly didn't know. She might have approved, but at age nineteen, I did not want to discuss my sex life with my mother.

I dressed and walked to the front desk to pay for the wasted appointment. When the office nurse intercepted me with a prescription for a one-year supply of Enovid, I was as stunned as I was relieved.

Given my fierce determination to avoid pregnancy, I couldn't imagine anyone being more than a month or two pregnant when she came for an abortion. Clearly, such a person was irresponsible—or doing something wrong.

That self-centered point of view lasted about two weeks into my employment at the Fairmount Center. I was brand-new to the realities of providing abortions. We had no sonography, and we made appointments by phone based on the patient's request to terminate her pregnancy and her menstrual history. All of our patients were, by date of last normal menses, within the first trimester of pregnancy. We calculated gestation with the same slim cardboard calendar wheels that obstetricians used to estimate due dates and plan deliveries. Abortion clinics all over the United States had those wheels printed with the name of the abortion clinic, not an obstetrical service, as a symbol of "women's freedom of choice." Pregnancy was no longer synonymous with childbearing—unless you were "too far along."

The first time I had to turn a patient away because she was "too far along" is what did it for me.

I held the young woman's hand as she chanted through her sobs, "What will I do? What will I do?" She was lying on the surgery table, already gowned for the abortion she could not have. I had counseled the woman, so I knew she was not prepared to have a child. She was in college, on a birth control pill, and she and her boyfriend were both headed to law school. They had no wish to start a family now—education and a career came first. She didn't want to sacrifice her dreams and couldn't imagine derailing his career. When she missed her period, they had both prayed and waited for her next menstrual cycle. Surely she was not pregnant—she was on the pill. When she missed a second period, she'd gone to the school infirmary for a pregnancy test. It was positive, and the school nurse had referred her to us.

Following our counseling session, she had met the doctor, signed the medical consent form, and then undressed for the procedure. I was learning to perform pelvic exams to estimate the size of the pregnancy, and I still remember the doctor teaching me: "Walnut, lemon, orange, grapefruit. If it's a walnut, she may be too early. If you feel a grapefruit, warn me because she may be too far gone." I had felt a grapefruit, a large one, and hoped I was wrong.

Now I had no solution to offer, no place to refer the patient other than Hope Cottage, a Dallas "home for unwed mothers," to use the language of the time. I helped her dress, walked her to the door, and returned to the procedure room to cry in private while cleaning the room for the next patient.

As I continued my day's work, the distraught patient haunted me. My response was emotional: forcing a woman to continue a pregnancy—for any reason, including being later in the pregnancy—felt wrong. My prejudice had been washed away with tears for a real person, one with whom I could easily identify. Now I wondered: What did I really think and feel about abortion later in pregnancy?

In 1974, I knew little about fetal development and even less about the medical risks that came with advancing gestation. Like most people, I had no idea that pregnancy, labor, and delivery all carry greater risks to the life and health of the woman than abortion. But by the time of our return to Dallas in 1978, as Curtis was developing techniques to safely terminate pregnancy further and further into the second trimester, I needed to educate myself so I could be responsive to the needs of our patients and staff. Above all—and this part is no small thing—I needed to feel confident that I was on solid moral ground.

Once again, I would learn the most profound lesson from our patients.

I had imagined that patients would be both curious and concerned about the fetus as well as the increased medical risk they were taking when facing a later-term pregnancy. I ordered every book available with drawings or photos of the developing fetus, and I worked with the CDC's Abortion Surveillance System team to keep our information about risks up to date. It turned out that those were my big concerns, not our patients'. They were not interested in the photos and drawings, and few had any concept of relative risk. Patients at twenty-two weeks were worried about the same things patients worried about at six weeks: How much will the abortion cost? Will it hurt? When can I return to my normal life?

I was surprised—at first. However, I was not only a care provider but (like everyone else) sometimes a patient too. At about this same time, I needed dental surgery. My dentist knew I was interested in all things medical, so he explained the procedure to me in great detail. As I left his office to prepare for surgery the following day, I was grateful that he had the technical details down, but they were his responsibility, not mine.

I know far too much about this, I thought. *All I really care about is how long the surgery will take, how much it will hurt, and when I can eat again.*

Ah-ha! Suddenly I understood our own patients' point of view.

However, a deeper lesson had been with me far longer, and I am continually reminded of it by the nightly news: Some pregnancies are cherished babies before they are ever conceived, and tragically some pregnancies are not—even after they are delivered. Babies left in dumpsters make the second point, as do endless stories of child abuse and neglect. At the opposite pole, anyone who has longed to have a child knows the power of the imagined baby. Friends taught me this lesson when I was still in graduate school. After trying to conceive for over a year and finally getting pregnant, they decided on an outrageous male moniker: Giuseppi Luigi Piazzola. When their beautiful little girl was born, they were overjoyed . . . yet curiously disappointed. In gaining their longed-for child, they had lost the imaginary boy with the wonderful name.

To this day, when I hear Frank Sinatra's poignant song from *Carousel*, "My Boy Bill," I'm hooked. As the song opens, I take offense at the blatant sexism in the impending father's wish to raise a rascal son who'll chase the girls. Then I'm touched by the singer's disorientation when he registers that his child might be a girl, and his determination to protect a daughter from just the sort of boy he'd imagined. Indeed, the meaning of each pregnancy rests in the hopes and dreams and fears of the parents.

Gestational age is only one factor in whether a pregnancy is welcome news, and usually not the most important to patients—nor, as I would repeatedly learn, to me. The quality of life in store for each pregnancy—the risk versus benefit, the anticipated burden or joy—is what drives most patients' decisions, and that is a calculation only the pregnant woman is qualified to make.

But getting to that clarity has been a journey for me. My own journey gives me patience with our staff as they navigate their inner worlds of meaning—surrounding pregnancy, fetal development, childbearing, and ultimately life.

Just as we never want patients to take soul-harming action, we would never ask a staff member to do soul-harming work. As the clinic increased its gestational limits, some staff struggled. Our staff are like many (perhaps most) people: the more the developing pregnancy resembles a baby, the more feelings it arouses. For most of our staff, although their commitment to the availability of safe, legal abortion doesn't waver, they learn through experience what level of participation they can and cannot manage for themselves. This line in the sand is intellectual and emotional and sensual—sights and sounds and smells are also at play.

Some staff have needed a change in role, usually shifting to office work. Others have needed to move on altogether. Those who stayed would continue their personal journey in monthly staff meetings, in private conversations with their supervisor, and with each other. Ignoring our feelings doesn't work. Exploring those feelings with the understanding and support of colleagues allows us to go on in good conscience and to provide similar support to our patients. We are all asking questions to which there are no absolute right or wrong answers—only our own best answers at the time.

Events in our own lives, both past and present, are often an overriding factor. For years I worked with a physician who was deeply committed to providing abortions. At the same time, she and her husband struggled to conceive. With fertility treatment, they were able to have twins—a happy outcome for all. When she returned to the work she loved, she set a firm gestational limit of twelve weeks and, with goodwill, referred patients who were farther in their pregnancies to other doctors. She had the emotional maturity and the professionalism to distinguish her own experience and its emotional impact from the needs of patients—and still find a way to take care of herself and her patients.

. . . .

Creating healthy ways to manage our own feelings about fetal bodies is an ongoing process for many of our staff. I have always believed that an awareness of our mixed and evolving feelings can allow greater appreciation of the wide range of feelings about abortion that patients present.

For patients, confusion and conflicting feelings can be a problem at any point in gestation. For most staff members, who are clear in their intellectual commitment to abortion rights, it's the sensory elements of abortion later in pregnancy that can throw their abstract commitment into question: *How can abortion be right if it makes me feel queasy?* This reexamination of our beliefs and values not only aids our own moral development but can also improve our patient care.

I learned this deeply personal lesson in 1979. Our home phone rang in the middle of the night; it was Daniece, the nurse on call. Curtis had inserted laminaria for a fourteen-year-old patient earlier in the day and then sent her home with her mother and instructions to return the following day to complete her abortion. Her mother, Jackie, had called Daniece, sounding near panic as she described her daughter, Amy.

"She's in pain like she's never had before," the worried mother reported. "And when I took her to the bathroom, there was so much blood. I'm scared!"

Daniece believed Amy was essentially in labor, induced by the laminaria, and instructed Jackie to drive from their home directly to the clinic where we would meet them.

Curtis and I drove the few blocks from our home to the office. The moon was full, and I was enchanted by the glowing suburban landscape—the bare branches of huge sycamore trees lining the streets were golden in the light. We met Daniece as she unlocked the back door.

While she set up the procedure room, Curtis and I found mother and daughter huddled at our front door.

Curtis swiftly moved Amy, swaddled in a blanket from home, to the prepared room. As I took Jackie to our patient recovery room, she continued the story she'd begun with Daniece, explaining, "It was as if she were in labor, and I had so wanted to spare her that pain." So had we.

By the time I entered the procedure room, Amy was holding Daniece's arm, pulling her close, saying, "Thank you! Thank you for making the pain stop."

Curtis was standing at the foot of the exam table, holding the intact fetus Amy's body had just efficiently expelled before slipping it into a stainless-steel basin. He had the sad gaze I often saw when he performed a second-trimester abortion, and his gentleness with the fetus seemed almost loving to my eyes. Then I took the basin, and he shifted his full attention to carefully suctioning Amy's uterus to remove the placenta and ensure that her bleeding was minimal.

At the time, we were donating all tissue from abortions after fifteen weeks to Southwestern Medical School, where research on lung development would eventually allow medicine to accelerate fetal lung maturation for women at risk of losing their pregnancies to preterm labor and delivery.

For many of our patients this was an unexpected silver lining in their abortion decision—a way to give other women, whose circumstances were different from their own, the hope of keeping their premature births alive at earlier gestations than had ever been possible.

It was a perfect nineteen-week fetus.

With my right hand, I transferred the fetus into one of the labeled cups and popped the lid tight. It had been warm, still Amy's body temperature, and it was so small that it nested in the palm of my hand. The thin membrane that would have become its many-layered skin was delicate, translucent. I had been fascinated by fetal development since my first encounter with such a specimen in a biology lab, so I disciplined my curious mind and quickly placed the sealed container in the lab refrigerator.

I had a patient to return to. I stepped back into the procedure room to help Amy into her pajamas and walked her to meet her mother.

As I sat on the bench at the head of the procedure room hallway to allow Amy and Jackie a moment of privacy, I overheard them in the adjacent recovery room. Amy told her mother how easy it had been once we'd taken charge, and how glad she would be to go back to school. Jackie murmured her love, saying, "I'm so proud of you. You were so brave."

They chatted as mother and daughter but also as friends.

I could still feel the soft, warm fetus in my palm, and I caught myself thinking, *They could have had a baby. It would have been born into such a loving family, and they have the money to make it work.* So many of our patients lack those advantages.

We had dimmed the hallway lights. Daniece had cleaned the room and gone home. Curtis was completing the patient chart as we waited thirty minutes for a final bleeding check. Alone in the quiet, darkened space, I was fully identified with the fetus I had held. I shook my head, and perhaps it was my own mother's voice, always reasonable, that echoed in my head: *Glenna, she's only fourteen—a child herself. She has her whole life ahead. Is it really the time for her to have a baby?*

That voice called me back to reality—Amy's reality.

That long moment in the dark increased my sympathy for patients who struggle with conflicting beliefs and feelings. It has also given me a reservoir of patience with our staff when they are thrown off by unexpected feelings and perhaps even some insight into the fervent opposition to abortion rights.

In my experience with abortion, political rhetoric provides no useful guidance. Those who rabidly oppose legal abortion accuse us of "murder," while many abortion advocates want us to dismiss the significance of the fetus. The potential of the fetus is far more visible in later-term abortion, and for both Curtis and me, it does hold value. As providers, we want to honor the fetus *and* be at peace with the end of that fetal life. For each of us, coming to terms with the complexity of our work is an ongoing process.

By any measure, this journey has helped me feel enriched by my work and more committed to each woman's right to decide the fate of her pregnancy. Ever since that soul-searching moment in the dark, I've understood the deep tension in our work and known that abortion is truly a forced choice between a life already in the midst of living and a potential life. Within that transcendent moment, I felt disembodied, suspended in the moonlit sky of our drive through the sycamore trees, and I knew that our lives, filled with endless decisions, are precious, glowing things.

The power of that experience defies words—even my own.

. . . .

Dealing with a larger fetus was not the only challenge our staff faced as we saw more patients who were further in their pregnancies. Addressing medical risks and handling patients' pain were the other chief worries. Curtis was focused on patient safety, and his concern was evident in the ever-changing medical protocols, so patients were covered in that area. What we all needed now was more effective pain management.

So, I turned my focus to the more elusive elements of physical pain. The first thing I did was observe our counselors at work in the procedure rooms. I wanted to applaud the good work they were already doing and learn from their missteps. Much of what I saw confirmed my assumptions about how to handle pain—that a calm demeanor and quiet tone of voice, combined with close attention to nonverbal cues from the patient, were essential—but one observation shook me to the core of my feminist biases.

I silently entered the room as the counselor dimmed the lights, turned on soft music, and helped the patient into the leg rests. I knew from her chart that she was a twenty-year-old college student. Stepping briefly to the head of the table, I introduced myself and let her know that I would be in the room with her counselor, watching over her. The patient smiled as the counselor quietly told her that the doctor was about to begin the procedure, but at the doctor's first touch, the young woman moaned as if in pain.

Soon she was whimpering like a frightened child, jerking away each time the doctor attempted to insert the speculum. She pulled her legs from the rests and curled into a fetal position on the table. The doctor—a friendly, easygoing OB-GYN resident who was finishing his training at the Catholic hospital near the clinic—simply put down his instruments and waited. Then the counselor began to coo and hum, repeating phrases in what sounded like baby talk.

I was appalled. Our mission was women's empowerment. This counselor was infantilizing the patient, and it was insulting.

It was also working.

Using baby talk, the counselor was able to coax the patient from her fetal position back into the leg rests, and, still cooing the words, the counselor repeated, "Now the doctor will touch you."

The soothed "child" on the table allowed the doctor to go to work, and her procedure was complete in minutes. When the patient sat up and began to dress, she had only one question: "Where can I get something for lunch? I'm starving." She spoke in an adult voice—as if nothing out of the ordinary had occurred.

I took note. The counselor had fallen back on her experience as a mother of three small children, but I realized she had done what good therapists and—as we would learn—hypnotists do: she met the patient where she was. The counselor made emotional contact with the patient's frightened inner child and, mimicking the patient's own sounds, gently guided the young woman toward a more mature way of coping.

Fascinated, I did what my mother had taught me to do: I went to the library and searched the literature. That's when I found the groundbreaking work of psychiatrist Milton Erickson. Erickson struggled throughout his life with pain and physical limitations from polio he'd contracted at age seventeen. Against medical odds, he had survived, but he was unable to move or speak for months. As a teenager, he'd taught himself to speak and, with the aid of a cane, walk again, all through positive self-talk and concentration on muscle memory. Essentially, he recovered through self-hypnosis.

As a psychiatrist, Erickson was particularly influential in the 1960s and 1970s, drawing on his experience to develop a form of hypnotherapy that was interactive and collaborative, with the patient as a full participant. His approach to "medical hypnosis" mirrored our wish for patients to feel that they had control over their abortion experience. So, in the late 1970s, Curtis and I attended a meeting of the organization he founded: the American Society of Clinical Hypnosis.

I expected the flower children of medicine. Instead, we encountered four hundred other medical doctors—what today we would call the "old White men" of medicine—plus one other woman and one other psychologist. There were anesthesiologists who wanted to use "positive suggestion" to limit the toxic drugs of their trade but also men from all fields who recognized the power of the mind-body connection. Medical hypnosis for pain management, I soon learned, was not a fringe movement in mainstream medicine. Bill Moyers, the noted TV journalist, would go on to capture the tenor of the times (as he often did) in his 1993 TV series and subsequent bestselling book *Healing and the Mind*.

Medically, we were in good company. However, we encountered resistance from our staff when we started adding "skills in hypnosis" to their job descriptions. The word conjured an image of carnival sideshow hucksters in top hat and tails, waving a pocket watch while instructing audience members to quack like a duck or otherwise embarrass themselves in public. So we took a lesson from Erickson and dropped the word "hypnosis." Instead, we schooled our staff to think of everything they said and did—from tone of voice to hand gestures—as affecting the mood state and medical outcome of our patients.

We created simple but effective rules: *Always gently knock on a door before entering a patient's room. Make eye contact when talking. Close doors quietly. Dim lights when possible.* Hypnosis is not about manipulation but about focus, being present in the moment, meeting the patient where she is, and guiding her—with her permission and participation—toward a more relaxed state. In fact, we called it "relaxation," and we practiced what we preached.

At the end of every staff meeting, Curtis or I led the staff in a guided meditation. Some days, we imagined a walk in the woods or a day at the beach. In other sessions, we led the group in a body scan, guiding their attention from feet to ankles to shins, moving all the way up to the crown of the head, inviting each part of the body to relax. Such techniques are commonplace today, but in the late 1970s their use in medicine was innovative and often met with skepticism. Our medical director, Dr. John Armstead, an excellent technician and former professional athlete—he'd put himself through medical school playing for the Harlem Globetrotters summer team—had his doubts. But as the staff became fluent in guiding patients to relax during the procedure, he declared, "I like it. Patients do have less pain, and that makes me feel good."

We had full staff support, and patients were experiencing a significant improvement in their care.

We have always used patient feedback forms—*How did the abortion compare with what you expected? What was the most difficult part? What do you wish we had done differently?*—and shared that feedback with the staff. With the addition of medical hypnosis to our care, patients consistently told us that the abortion was so much easier than they had expected, that it was over before they knew it. We'd come to expect such comments from patients in the first trimester, but now we were getting identical feedback from our second-trimester patients—despite the longer procedure time. We also had fewer reports of post-op pain and fewer anxious calls from patients in the days following their abortion. Patients were happier, and our staff took pride in their second-trimester abortion care.

We had achieved our goal and were excited to share what we'd learned. I later wrote about our work in two medical textbooks.[15] My contribution was aptly titled "Nonpharmacological Pain Management" and described individual counseling to establish rapport and prepare the patient for the procedure, as well as the use of positive suggestion, relaxation, and guided imagery during the abortion. When we spoke at professional meetings about our multilayered approach to pain management, however, our words made it sound too complicated and time consuming. Finally we made a video of our virtually painless procedures. Doctors and administrators could see that the simple interventions we built into our work with every patient paid off—and with little or no increase in time or cost.

Sometimes seeing is believing.

. . . .

My perpetual quest to promote well-being among both patients and staff renewed my interest in "burnout." The term had emerged in popular culture and the social sciences just as Curtis and I were taking our much-needed respite in the mountains. Then my interest had felt personal; now it was professional. I wanted to help our staff avoid burnout, which was becoming a catchphrase in the helping professions and, in my mind, dovetailed with the issues raised as we increased our second-trimester abortion service.

Feelings about the fetus, fear of serious medical complications, and the difficulty of witnessing patients in pain are all potential sources of wear and tear on staff, often leading to "compassion fatigue"—one of the formal definitions of burnout. In burnout, we shut down our own feelings and, thus, shut down our compassion for the feelings of others. Unacknowledged confusion, fear, and a sense of failure then leave us inordinately fatigued, easily frustrated, quick to direct anger and blame at others, and cynical about our patients and our work.

None of us are immune to accumulated work stress—I've known too many burned-out psychotherapists to think anyone is exempt. So, back to the library I went.

I devoured the literature on burnout, leaning into our professional responsibility to cultivate an ever-stronger connection to the social and moral values that originally drew us to the work.[16] Doing good in the world and doing it well are lofty ideals but have to be tempered by experience. Otherwise, we are bound to fall short, especially in our own eyes—making us our own proverbial worst enemy. This is why good supervision on the job and a supportive team of coworkers is critical. With proactive support, naive idealism can mature into realistic expectations that allow us to enjoy our successes and learn from all the rest.

I found ways to use this fresh perspective in monthly training and supervision for our staff, who appreciated the attention to their needs. Also important was learning that they were not alone—that other dedicated workers in a variety of human services, from psychology and medicine to teaching and law enforcement (not to mention housewives), also struggle with exhaustion, loss of idealism, and fears of failure.[17] The concept of burnout had captured my interest not only because I wanted to nurture our staff but because the characteristics of those most vulnerable to burnout—youth, idealism, ambition—were qualities I looked for in employees and valued in myself.

Colleagues across the country heard about the burnout workshops I was developing and asked me to do one at the NAF Annual Meeting in New York City in 1979 at The Essex House overlooking Central Park. I had expected to facilitate a small group therapy session in a meeting room; instead I had to push my way through a standing-room-only crowd with people spilling into the hallway. I was terrified. Fortunately, I had overprepared and, stepping up to the microphone provided by a resourceful NAF staffer, I spoke from my copious notes—a lecture, not a discussion. Adrenaline conquered my fear, and I got through the meeting.

Grateful and exhausted when it was over, I returned to Dallas—only to learn that it wasn't over.

NAF meetings were still open forums then, with little to no security, and the organization, in its commitment to public education about abortion, had provided the New York Times with an advance copy of the Annual Meeting program. In the week before the meeting, a Times reporter had called me at home—our phone number was still listed, though in the years to come the FBI and DOJ would advise us to unlist all our personal information—and grilled me about the "high rate" of burnout in abortion clinics. She provoked me to a heated rebuttal of the anti-abortion assertion that "killing babies every day" was the cause of staff burnout. If burnout wasn't rampant, she reasoned, why was I even on the program?

Inexperienced with major media outlets, I decided to get rid of her by faxing her my working notes—surely she'd be bored with my low-key tone and academic references. When I did not see her at the meeting, I thought my ploy had worked. Instead, her story appeared on the front page of the Style section of the Friday Times on July 20, 1979. Within the headline story, "Abortion Rights in Peril, Say Advocates at Conference," was a sidebar on my workshop titled "Clinic Staffers Suffer Emotional Traumas Too."

Although the sidebar's text was faithful to my working notes, the title and context were not. The larger article described the NAF Annual Meeting as "a call to battle" against growing political opposition to abortion rights; it cast abortion advocates as "on the defensive" on this "burning issue." When the journalist directly quoted my rebuttal, "I do not believe I am a baby killer," I *sounded* defensive. Damn. Plus, it was placed directly above an article titled "A Clothes Emporium with a Surplus of Whimsy," complete with a photo collage of fancifully dressed young New Yorkers on the street and shelves overflowing with hats. Later, I would find the whole experience ironic—Was abortion a burning social and political issue or a bit of fashion whimsy? At the time I felt trivialized.

The NAF Hotline—designed to respond to callers with information, consultation, and referrals—was on fire with calls from member clinics. According to Dr. Uta Landy, the executive director, half of the callers were outraged that I had dared to "air our dirty laundry" about burnout. The other half wanted me to do a workshop at their NAF facilities. While I was feeling misrepresented and misunderstood, Uta recognized the opportunity. There was "good work" to do, and Uta wanted to do it with me.

Together, we spent the next several years doing burnout workshops for member clinics all over the United States. This gratifying work connected both of us with dedicated staff in a variety of work settings: hospitals, doctors' offices, and clinics, both large and small. Our emphasis on the self-care and the institutional nurturing required to maintain staff energy and idealism was especially timely as the social and political environment was growing more hostile to women and abortion.

The *New York Times* coverage had, of course, ignored the good I was trying to do and instead played on those growing hostilities. I had a lot to learn about dealing with the media. Sadly, I would have many future opportunities to do so.

CHAPTER SEVEN

Tumultuous Times: Living with What We Cannot Understand

"Today was a day I never saw coming. No where in my life did I
ever think I'd be here making one of the toughest decisions in my life,
but I myself know what will be the best for me as much as it hurts. I
know I'll recover from this and move on. I'll now know how hard it is to
go through something that you never see coming. I know I'll always live
with this guilt but I pray to my savior to help me in life to continue."
—*Patient journal entry*

Curtis

It was the seventh anniversary of *Roe v. Wade*, Tuesday, January 22,
1980—a date that had changed my life and, more importantly, the lives
of all women in America. I certainly did not see what was coming.

The previous day in our Dallas clinic I'd met a devoted young couple—devoted to each other, to their fifteen-month-old baby, and to
their faith. I read the essential facts on the cover sheet of the patient's
medical record: Angela was twenty-two years old, this was her second
pregnancy, and our sonogram revealed that she was now sixteen weeks

pregnant. Her husband, Thomas, held their sleeping baby in his arms as they explained their situation.

Thomas was the assistant pastor of the African Baptist Church in a small Texas town much like the Athens of my childhood. Angela had a college education and worked at the day care center affiliated with the church—which allowed her to both care for their baby and pursue her career interest in early childhood education. Their life was full—nearly overfull. Their birth control method had failed, and although they wanted more children in the future, this was not the right time.

We signed the consent forms together and, as part one of the two-step procedure, I inserted laminaria. The family spent the night in a motel nearby while the laminaria tents did their work.

Tuesday morning at 8:30, Angela returned for her D&E. We proceeded as usual: The counselor set up the surgery tray and dimmed the lights. The nurse started an IV and administered pain medications. Angela and the counselor chatted in soothing tones. I let the patient know I was in the room by gently touching her knee.

"I am here now," I said softly. "Just continue to relax."

I began the procedure as I always did, removing the laminaria and gently inserting metal dilators, each slightly larger than the last, to open the patient's softened cervix just enough to complete the evacuation. The process was going smoothly when she suddenly stiffened, then jerked. I heard gasping. The counselor called, "Dr. Boyd, she's not breathing!"

I moved to the head of the table. Angela was still. She had no pulse. She was in cardiac arrest.

The counselor turned on the emergency call light, and Brenda, our head nurse, rushed in. Brenda and I began CPR while another nurse called 911. To our relief, Angela started to breathe on her own. Her pulse was thready but present.

Our relief was short-lived. Within minutes she suffered a second cardiac arrest. The paramedics had arrived and took over the second resuscitation. When Angela's heartbeat resumed and her blood pressure stabilized, the paramedics were able to transport her to Parkland Hospital.

I called the emergency room at Parkland to talk with the chief resident—a professional courtesy, but in this case, I wanted to convey the urgency I felt. This patient had suffered two cardiac arrests with no apparent cause.

I then spoke briefly with Thomas, who naturally was frightened and confused. The counselor who had been with Angela accompanied him to the hospital—our standard procedure. She and Thomas alternated walking the baby while they waited, as we all did, for news on Angela's condition.

Glenna went into action as well. As she later told me, her first thought was for the patients and families sitting in the waiting room. Having heard the sirens and seen the uniformed paramedics walking our hallway, they had to be worried. Glenna calmly introduced herself and explained that we had transported a patient to the hospital, that her family had been notified immediately and had accompanied her. Medical transport was always unnerving when it happened, she explained, but routine when we had concerns for a patient's safety.

Glenna held up one of our consent for surgery forms, noting that although the listed complications are rare, they are real, and one had happened. Then she invited patients and their families to ask any questions. Only one older man—perhaps the father of a patient—had asked, in a trembling voice, "You all do surgery here?" Like many people, he saw abortion as such a routine procedure that in his mind, it barely qualified as surgery. On an average day, his naive perspective was close to the truth.

"Yes," Glenna replied in her calmest tone. "The abortion is technically a minor surgery."

She reassured the silent room that each patient would meet privately with a counselor and that we would meet with any family member who wished. They could ask questions at that time as well, and if they preferred, they could reschedule. Every patient stayed to have her abortion, and I stayed to perform those abortions. I did so as I have always done—carefully, methodically. Yet I was more keenly aware of my every move, as if a part of me were watching over my own shoulder.

When we took our lunch break, Glenna and I walked to our nearby condo. It was a cool, sunny winter's day, and birds chirped in the bare branches of the trees, reminding me of a world beyond the clinic walls. At home, I lay down on the sofa with my head in Glenna's lap. I felt cold, a bone-deep chill I'd never felt before. Glenna wrapped me in a blanket and heated some soup. We forced ourselves to eat before returning to the clinic for a full afternoon of surgical patients.

Between procedures, I went to the staff lounge to make and receive calls from the hospital. Our staff gathered around to listen. The updates were not encouraging. At about 1:30, the counselor called from the hospital to talk with Glenna. Angela was bleeding internally. The emergency room physicians had done everything they could, but they could not stop the bleeding. Angela was dying.

Glenna told me privately, and then she told the rest of the staff. We all took a break to let the news sink in. Feeling numb, I retreated to an empty surgery room to sit alone. Glenna lingered in the front office to be nearby as staff hugged and cried, squeezed each other's hands, and patted each other's shoulders. Somehow, we all carried on. The afternoon patients needed our care.

Glenna also made all the necessary phone calls. She called the National Abortion Federation leadership, the other abortion providers in Dallas, our insurance company, and our attorney. She called the Centers for Disease Control to report the death and the Dallas County Medical Examiner's Office to request an autopsy. She wanted them to hear the news from us—as an act of respect, but she also wanted their expert guidance. She called everyone she thought would need to know, but she did not call anyone in the media. We knew that we would have to address the media at some point, but we didn't yet know enough about what happened to make a responsible public statement.

That night, Glenna dreamed that a crowd of angry people beat her around the head and shoulders with rolled-up newspapers. She couldn't read the headline, but she knew it had to be about the patient's death. It made sense that her nightmare featured the media. Since her experience with the *New York Times*, media coverage had only become more inflammatory.

We would soon learn the hard way not to wait for the media to come to us.

. . . .

Caring for our staff was our top priority. Fortunately, we had an in-service staff meeting already scheduled for the next day, January 23. We gathered in a private conference room at the Stoneleigh Hotel, across the street from the clinic, and we used the time and space to process what had happened.

I had no words, but I knew others would need to talk. It was painful but necessary work, and I was grateful that Glenna could lead us. She asked everyone to share the first thing they had done after arriving home the night before, and she began that conversation with a confession: she had called her mother and sworn her to secrecy, and they had cried together. That brought the whole staff to tears, and words began to flow. Most of them had also called their own mother, each imagining that she was the only one.

Then Glenna asked everyone—me included—to write anonymously about the patient's death. She gave us places to start.

The hardest part for me was . . .

What I wish had been done differently was . . .

What helped me most was . . .

I don't remember what I wrote, or even if I wrote. Looking back, I can't imagine how heavy that pen must have felt in my hand. But the staff embraced the task. They shared some of what they had written:

"What helped me most was being able to talk about it with the rest of the staff."

"Verbalizing and generating ideas of what to do next was the most therapeutic for me."

"What helped me most was talking with staff at the Stoneleigh and seeing the emotions of Curtis and his genuine care for each patient."

This last comment touched me deeply. Like everyone else gathered in our circle, I felt raw and so very protective of our staff.

Suddenly, in the middle of our intimate conversation, the swinging doors to the room flew open, and in stormed a woman holding a microphone, a man holding lights, and another man with a TV news camera—Channel 4 FOX News. The tape was rolling. It was Glenna's nightmare manifest. "We have information that a woman who came to you for an abortion was killed at your clinic yesterday!" the woman shouted. "We have some questions."

My grief and sadness turned to rage. I leapt to my feet. "This is a private meeting," I roared. "You are not invited. Get out, out, out!" Clearly, I was not the right person to deal with the media.

The media, Glenna would later remind me, is not necessarily the enemy. It's easy to make negative assumptions about their motives, just as it's easy for them to assume the worst about us—and this reporter certainly seemed to. But ultimately, news reporters want the truth, just as we do.

Glenna ushered the news team out the door, but she recognized the need to address their questions. The staff, too, understood the weight of the moment. "Go on. You can do it," they encouraged as she stepped into the hall. "It will be OK." I know she would have liked time to gather her thoughts, but there was no time.

The staff gathered around the door to eavesdrop. So did I. I was impressed by Glenna's calm in the face of those bright lights and the barrage of questions. Between questions, interruptions, and accusations, she managed to state our concerns:

Yes, a patient of ours died in Parkland Hospital yesterday. We do not know the cause of death. We also want to know. We have requested an autopsy. We have notified the Office of the Medical Examiner and the CDC. Please contact them. Abortion-related deaths are rare. This death is our first, and it is of grave concern to us also. We must maintain confidentiality for our patient and her family. And we are concerned about distorted and adverse publicity about this death, as that has consequences for the

whole abortion movement and the availability of a much-needed service.
This is a potentially explosive issue. Clearly, that is why you are here.
We will not engage in speculation. We will share accurate information as
soon as we have it. Please do not use the patient's name on the air.[18]

This unexpected interview was on the evening news. There was Glenna, looking strained, as the news woman's voiceover reported the death, cited CDC statistics on abortion mortality, and noted that this was our first death in over fifty thousand abortions performed at our clinic since 1973. Although Glenna was never quoted, under duress she had distilled the salient points and set the tone. The newswoman used the facts, but despite Glenna's plea, she also used the patient's name. Given the patient and her husband's concern for confidentiality, this was particularly disturbing to us.

Glenna and I decided to hold our own press conference at the clinic that very night. To draft a press release, we called the medical examiner for an update and received permission to release preliminary results from the autopsy. Only two reporters attended: one from each of the Dallas newspapers. Most of our staff came—at 8:00 p.m. after a long and difficult day—as a show of support. In keeping with Glenna's earlier impromptu statements, we told the reporters what we knew and what we did not. We answered questions. Afterward, each reporter asked to use our phone to update their editors: *No news here.*

This was a relief.

A second TV news installment included an interview with the be-reaved husband in his mother's living room. He kept repeating, "I don't understand. I just don't understand why."

By Friday night, Channel 4 was making unsubstantiated charges—suggesting that the death was due to error or neglect. Only one newspa-per, *The Dallas Morning News*, picked up the story. The piece was short, appearing on pages 18 and 43, and reported the patient's death in the larger context of contemporary medical care and informed consent.

The following week, the medical examiner determined that the cause of death was disseminated intravascular coagulopathy, or DIC, "due to amniotic fluid embolism due to medical abortion."[19] In lay terms: The fluid in which the developing pregnancy floats had entered the patient's bloodstream. Bubbles had traveled to her lungs and heart, causing respiratory and cardiac arrest. The respiratory and cardiac arrest occurred on my surgery table, but what proved fatal was the fluid contents' interaction with the blood, which virtually eliminated the body's natural clotting response. That was why her bleeding could not be stopped. The report concluded: "Manner of death—accident."

When the medical examiner's report came out, our clinic issued another press release. There was no media coverage. From a journalistic perspective, it was not newsworthy.

As we would learn from the CDC, DIC is extremely rare, unforeseeable, and unpreventable. It is more likely to occur during childbirth than with abortion. I suppose this should have made me feel better: I had done nothing wrong. But I took little comfort.

· · · ·

Even now, years later, I'm not sure I understand how devastated I was by our patient's death. Angela was young, healthy, and early enough in her pregnancy that I had felt neither apprehension nor premonition as I began her procedure. She'd expressed no worries of her own other than keeping the abortion a secret from her family and their church. I certainly understood and even identified with that concern.

I had liked Angela and been confident that I could care for her safely, so I was caught off guard when her heart stopped beating on my surgery table. It had seemed unreal, yet once it happened, I had known that something was very wrong. I had sensed then that she would die.

As a doctor I was trained to manage crises, to always think of the patient's welfare, not my own. Through all the years I provided illegal abortions, a patient death had been my worst fear. Those years of fear were an additional load on my heart and mind—one I could not acknowledge because that fear had been for myself. So although I felt great sadness for Angela and her family, I suspect there was another component: her death awakened those years of so many fears—for my career, my freedom, my family's well-being—that I did not want to remember. I had been so fortunate through my years of providing illegal abortions. Now that the procedure was legal—and Glenna and I had dedicated ourselves to making it as safe, as sensitive to patients' and their families' needs, and as available as possible—I was living my worst fear.

As a general practitioner back in Athens, I had lost patients. Most of them were older; some were parents or grandparents of my contemporaries. Most died of cancer or heart disease or simply old age. I did what I could to ease their suffering, and I grieved alongside their families, but those deaths were not surprises. Accidents and crib deaths were shocking, but I never became unmoored. This was different, and I was shaken.

Other abortion providers who have had a patient death have felt undone too—although I didn't learn this until later. Like me, nothing in their medical training or professional experience had prepared them for this particular situation. Abortion care is different from other medicine: it is a commitment to a social cause—women's liberation in general and reproductive justice in particular. It is nothing less than an effort to change women's place in society. With Angela's death, I felt that I had failed the greater cause.

I never lost confidence in my skills, but one of my sleepless nights produced a memory from medical school. A group of students were joking about becoming MDs—not medical doctors but "medical deities." Although it was lighthearted, this banter spoke to the attitude of some doctors at the time: convinced of their own invincibility in communities where they held power and respect. As a young man, I was far too serious about my religious beliefs, with their emphasis on humility, to join in. Now, Angela's death revealed a new dimension to the truth embedded in that joke. I had done nothing to cause her death, but it was set in motion on my surgery table. I'd had such confidence in my "magic hands" that I had taken my ability to manage technical challenges for granted. Yet I was no medical deity. I could not control Angela's fate—nor my own. Although I no longer spoke in the vocabulary of my religious youth, I was experiencing a "fall from grace."

I approach life and medicine as a series of puzzles to solve, and I solve them. The medical examiner's report essentially said that in this case, there was no puzzle to solve. Amniotic embolism is unforeseeable and unpreventable, and, when severe, its effects are unstoppable. I had been powerless. This, above all else, was unacceptable to me.

Like Millie, who wanted to prevent another patient's suicide, I wanted to prevent another patient's abortion-related death. To that end, I came up with a new protocol for D&E: rather than starting with dilation, I decided to begin the procedure by breaking the amniotic sac and draining the fluid before doing anything else, thus minimizing the opportunity for amniotic fluid to enter the bloodstream.

In the thousands of abortions we have provided since 1980, we have learned to recognize the subtle indicators of an amniotic fluid embolism (AFE)—sudden shortness of breath, an alteration in heartbeat or a drop in oxygen saturation level (both of which we measure continuously), sudden panic in a previously calm patient. Fortunately, most AFEs are minor and pass quickly—what medicine terms "sub-clinical." They do not progress to DIC. Still, we added this event to the list of medical risks in our consent form, and we are ever watchful.

I have never fully regained my sense of invulnerability. Perhaps this is for the best. As my early religious training taught me, pride goeth before a fall. The hypervigilance I lived with in my prelegal days returned, and Glenna and I created protocols for every known abortion-related complication. I didn't want to be taken unawares ever again.

What we did not foresee—although our experience with the media should have been a big clue—were the political complications outside our walls and beyond our control: the rise of the anti-abortion religious right.

. . . .

Of course, we knew that fundamentalist churches were growing—megachurches and TV evangelists were getting ample attention by the late 1970s. Minister and conservative activist Jerry Falwell was already a household name, but he had been railing mainly against desegregation. It was late in 1978 before he preached his first sermon against abortion, and the following year he founded the Moral Majority as a political action arm of White fundamentalist Christianity. Televangelists Jim and Tammy Faye Bakker were on the ascent too—not yet disgraced.

Neither Glenna nor I saw their opposition to abortion, grounded solely in their specific brand of Christianity, as a serious threat to the legal right to abortion. After all, mainstream conservative Christians were openly pro-choice: W. A. Criswell of the First Baptist Church of Dallas, who was then president of the Southern Baptist Conference, was on our side at first. So was the influential Reverend Billy Graham. We could not yet comprehend the rising tide of religious intolerance mingled with misogyny.

Time, and the swing of the political pendulum, would prove us wrong.

As we were taking this new age of women's empowerment for granted, the religious right had set its sights on abortion—a rallying crusade with even more money-making power than the evils of racial integration. Glenna, who has always been more attuned to the demonization of women than I, recognized that these religious crusaders saw abortion as the new scarlet letter—tapping into age-old beliefs about the dangers, even evil, of women's sexuality.[20] I thought she was exaggerating, but within the decade, clinics across the country were besieged by anti-abortion protesters damning women who sought abortions and the clinics providing them. Ours were not exempt.

These protestors operated without scruple. They carried posters featuring bloody deformed fetuses. They linked arms to create human walls to keep frightened patients away from the health services they needed. They knelt on our sidewalk to chant and pray. They invaded our clinic, knocking staff to the floor in order to chain themselves to exam tables and medical equipment. They gathered on our neighbor's property to get closer to our procedure rooms. Standing atop ladders, they yelled into megaphones in falsetto baby voices, "Mommy, don't kill me!"

At last, it became clear to us that a religious war on women's rights had begun.

We increased our own security measures—removing our names from the phonebook as the FBI and DOJ suggested and installing more sophisticated monitoring devices and alarms—but we stayed focused on caring for patients and staff. We warned patients when they made their appointments about the hostility they might face when entering the clinic. We pleaded with boyfriends and husbands and fathers not to respond to the bullying protestors. We spent extra counseling time with patients, letting them vent their pain and fury at the insults hurled at them as they walked to our door. We provided headphones with a guided meditation and soothing music while patients were in the surgery rooms. We brought in a psychologist who worked with staff to visualize imaginary shields for their emotional protection: *Step into your safety bubble as you walk to and from the clinic.*

Glenna used her perverse humor to dispel the tension, referring to the protesters as "our fans." They wanted attention, and they wanted to upset us, so she argued that our best strategy was to ignore them and their taunts. I agreed with her and lectured staff about not responding to the verbal abuse—and then lost my temper and screamed at the protest organizer as he followed Glenna and me to our car. So much for my good intentions.

On the whole, we adjusted to the constant hostile presence outside our doors. It became our new normal—until the harassment became truly violent. That Christmas Eve in 1988, when we were in Santa Fe with Kyle, anti-abortion vigilantes set fire to our Dallas clinic.

Glenna spent the night on the phone making travel arrangements, and we were on the first available flight back to Dallas. Neither of us had slept. The fog in my mind lifted as we walked through the blackened, waterlogged clinic. Two Methodist ministers had helped me buy that building—the first legal abortion facility in Texas—and now nameless, faceless "Christians" had tried to destroy it.

I was angry.

Although no one took credit for the arson, the federal Bureau of Alcohol, Tobacco and Firearms (BATF) agents who took over the case informed us that our fire had been set with the same rags and gasoline used to start suspicious fires at two other family planning facilities in Dallas. It wasn't just our absence from the clinic that made the timing ideal for the vigilantes. The arrival of the holidays meant the arsons were part of a larger pattern: Four people had been arrested in the first Christmas arson, in Pensacola, Florida, back in 1984.[21] As their attorney claimed, they were acting on the instructions of God—their named "coconspirator" in the court filings—to terrorize abortion clinics as a birthday present for Jesus.

My only thought was *I will not let them win!* I was determined to see patients in January as scheduled.

I got my wish because three people worked tirelessly. Lisa, our clinic director; Emerson, our financial officer; and Glenna got the job done.

Lisa returned early from the holiday with her rabidly anti-abortion in-laws, who had no idea of her work, to communicate with all staff, soothing their fears, so they would not learn of the arson from the evening news as she had.

Emerson worked with our insurance company to secure coverage of the building and furnishings, including the expensive medical equipment ruined by water damage.

Glenna dealt with the Dallas police and fire departments as well as the BATF agents in charge of the case. From her time as president of NAF a few years back, she had the regrettable advantage of past experience working with these organizations following clinic arsons and bombings. More importantly, she called a fire remediation company on Christmas day. We had no time to waste.

One of the firefighters had given Emerson a business card for a fire remediation company owned by a former firefighter. Although it was Christmas Day, Glenna called right away. A woman answered, and Glenna learned that it was a family business. The woman's husband called back first thing December 26. The entire family had been together for Christmas dinner, and all were eager to help. They started work just two days later, promising Glenna they could have us "ship shape" in time to open again.

"Our family is forever grateful that you were there for us when we needed you," one of the sons said to Glenna, pulling her aside in the wreckage. Both he and a brother had brought their girlfriends to us for abortions. "Now we're here for you."

Former patients called and volunteered to help in the clean-up too. While we didn't need any more help, both Glenna and I found it touching. Together, we got the job done.

On the morning of January 3, 1989, with a clear sense of triumph, we arrived in the clean, dry clinic to see our patients as scheduled. To our amazement and to Lisa's credit, not a single staff member quit as a result of the arson. Except for the folding chairs that filled in temporarily for sofas and chairs that could not be salvaged, it was eerily the same—as if nothing had happened and the arson had been a bad dream.

The arsonists were never identified, the crime was never solved, and I'm not sure I cared. What mattered most was that they could not stop us. We were open for business as usual. We were serving patients, and that was our ultimate goal.

CHAPTER EIGHT

No Time to Abandon Our Cause: The Decades of Violence

"All I ever wanted to be is a mother but I had to become a warrior to do so and at this point in my life I am tired of fighting. I felt today like I was taking the easy way out but thankfully I did it anyway. I am too damaged to have another baby when I am recovering from all the trauma custody battles can be especially when children are used as weapons. I thought my boyfriend loved me but today he didn't show up and when he finally was reached claimed it wasn't his baby. Ouch! I think I made the right choice because my 7 year old deserves my best and I obviously had to do some reevaluating my choices and start healing. Maybe a time not to be scrambling to barely get by but a time to rest take a deep breath and make changes. Perhaps this pregnancy was the illumination I needed to save my own life and be able to be there now and down the road for my boys."

—Patient journal entry

Glenna

Media analysts called the national tension around the abortion issue "explosive." Anti-abortion activists called it "war."[22] Unfortunately, by the mid-1980s, neither term was just a figure of speech. For us, the decade began with Angela's death and ended with our triumphant recovery from the Dallas arson. In the larger world, the 1980s introduced the most extreme harassment and violence against abortion facilities the United States had yet seen.

As president of the National Abortion Federation board of directors from May 1984 to June 1986, I presided over the organization through its most traumatic years to date. On July 4, 1984, the NAF offices in Washington, DC, were bombed in the night. I was unable to travel to Washington to speak at the press conference because I could not talk. I was recovering from major surgery for cancer after detecting a lesion at the base of my tongue in the week before my election and having surgery on Memorial Day.

Although I missed the news conference, I learned the meaning of terrorism—up close and personal. The FBI, in a 1983 report on domestic terrorist incidents, had defined terrorism as "the unlawful use of force or violence against persons or property to intimidate or coerce a government, the civilian population, or any segment thereof, in furtherance of political or social objectives."[23] In attacking the main provider organization, the perpetrators made their message clear: All abortion providers knew they could be next.

None of us felt safe. But in preparation for the media event I could not attend, I learned what NBC News coverage chose not to reveal: As the DC police and firefighters had picked through the debris of the NAF offices, they found a second, live pipe bomb, which the DC bomb squad later detonated in the nearby harbor. That bomb had contained enough TNT to level the entire block of office buildings and apartment houses. Families had been asleep in those apartments.

In the face of terrorism, no one is safe.

. . . .

In 1980 Ronald Reagan had garnered the Republican nomination and ultimately the election by creating a coalition of extremist factions within the Republican Party and disenfranchised Democrats. He was openly courting a new constituency that would soon become known as the religious right, a group galvanized by a shared fear of social change, especially the changing role of women in American society—embodied in the right to abortion.[24] The Republican platform promised a speedy end to legal abortion in the United States, with its support of a "human life" amendment to the Constitution and a plank advocating that federal judges be appointed on the basis of their anti-abortion opinions and rulings.

By the mid-1980s none of those promises had been fulfilled. Abortion remained legal, and women continued to have abortions at the same rate as before the start of the decade. Impatient, the most extreme elements within the anti-abortion movement grew disenchanted with legal means. Convinced that both the US president and God were on their side, they resorted to illegal methods.

From 1984 to 1986, US abortion providers sustained thirty-two arsons and forty-two bombings at a dollar cost of $10.3 million.[25] The emotional cost is impossible to calculate. Those events marked my years as NAF's president. Our 1988 arson in Dallas may have changed our lives forever, but it was simply one crime among many.

Then the ground shifted.

. . . .

After years of arsons and bombings, the 1990s became the decade of murder. The inflammatory language of the previous decade—labeling abortion as murder and abortion providers as murderers—became the justification for a series of killings. Doctors were the targets of choice, but receptionists, escorts, and security guards were also murdered— seven in total, plus another sixteen attempted murders in that decade alone, with more to come. And again, our lives would be forever changed by these events.

My first worry was for our staff. They were frightened, and many came under pressure from concerned family and friends to change careers. Few of them did, thankfully, but recruiting new staff became more difficult. Applicants had to consciously choose to work in the face of a clear and present danger that had not existed back when Curtis and I made our own commitment. I wondered if I would make that same choice again and suspected that I would. There was no way to know, but Kyle's pleading question—*Do you have to do this work?*—had not been an idle one.

Curtis's parents were in perpetual denial of his work and thus expressed no concern, but my parents worried for our safety. Curtis and I had serious, but abstract, conversations about closing the clinics and instead providing eldercare, as Curtis had in Athens before we met. We did not have to continue to provide abortions.

But the terrorism had a paradoxical effect on us: this was no time to abandon our cause.

· · · ·

Throughout the 1990s and the early 2000s, we also contended with increasing anti-abortion legislation and regulation at the state and federal levels. Our attorneys worked with pro-choice political groups to oppose and ameliorate those assaults on women's rights while we repeatedly adapted, making the best of things while doing whatever was required.

On January 1, 2004, the Texas Women's Right to Know Act (WRTK) went into effect. This law not only required us to "inform" every patient that abortion causes breast cancer, mental illness, and infertility—none of which is true—in the name of protecting women and their health, but it also required all abortions of sixteen weeks or more to be performed in a hospital or an ambulatory surgery center (ASC). Lying to patients was deeply disturbing—telling the truth is required by medical ethics—but women see through the patent disinformation campaign of WRTK laws.[26] Obeying the ASC requirements was far more onerous for patients and for us, doubling or tripling the cost of care.

Since our established clinic could not be retrofitted to meet ASC standards, we referred those patients to another Dallas facility that did meet the standards. We swallowed our business losses, taking comfort in knowing that women could still get care without unnecessary travel. We continued to see patients with a gestation of less than sixteen weeks at the Fairmount Center. Then, in 2007, the City of Dallas condemned that ASC's property for freeway expansion, putting them out of business. At that point we bought property and built our own surgery center in Dallas from the bottom up—but that decision came only after we'd suffered another major arson, this one at our other clinic in Albuquerque.

Again, the call came in the night—11:30 on Thursday, December 6, 2007. I fumbled in the dark and found the bedside phone: it was Joan, the director of our clinic in Albuquerque, New Mexico. She was speaking as if I'd entered a conversation already in progress. "It's burning, the entire building," she said. "The flames must be twenty—no, thirty feet high. Oh no! They're in the tree!" Joan's voice, always calm in crisis, became a wail. "Not the tree . . ."

When we arrived on the scene about forty-five minutes later, the flames were out. Molly, our director of nursing, was pacing the parking lot in her sweats and flip-flops. The firefighters, forty in all, swarmed the entire medical complex, looking for embers. They managed to save the tree and protect the other offices in our complex, but the destruction of our Albuquerque clinic was total.

Nineteen years had passed since the attack on our Dallas clinic, yet here we were again—the target of criminal rage and hostility.

I approached the fire chief in the front parking lot, hoping to get permission to enter the building and retrieve our appointment book—a white, plastic three-ring binder with *The Book* hand-lettered on the cover. This indispensable volume contained several weeks of patient appointments and contact information, and we needed to call the next day's patients. Unlike in Dallas, this arson occurred in the middle of a busy week; we had patients in the midst of multiday procedures who had to be seen, and staff scheduled for work with no place to go. We could not allow them to show up the next morning at a crime scene.

After entering the front office under police escort, I returned to the small group gathered around the fire chief and found that the owner of the complex had arrived. He introduced himself, saying that we'd been model tenants for twenty years and that he was pro-choice. He expressed his sympathy and assured me that we could rent an unoccupied unit while we rebuilt our own. I was grateful.

The next morning, staff gathered in Joan's scorched office. We used our personal cell phones to call patients, redirecting those whose immediate care was critical and rescheduling others. One of our doctors brought hospital-grade face masks for all of us, stressing the risks of smoke and chemical inhalation. With the help of a policeman, I entered the surgery area, and we picked our way through the mess of ash, sludge, and dripping water illuminated by his powerful flashlight. Electricity to our unit had been shut off in the night. Black holes marred the flooring where metal exam tables sagged, partially melted. A sink and its exposed plumbing lines draped down the walls in a grotesque parody of a Salvador Dali painting.

I fled the scene to tour the three available units, only to get a call from the owner with bad news: his property insurer now considered us too high a risk. Insurance coverage on all his US properties would be void if he allowed us to remain as tenants.

Our practice was homeless.

We gathered for a staff meeting in the home of our doctor, and Curtis asked the big question: "Do we want to continue with this work?"

"Tensions were high," one of our counselors, Amanda, subsequently told an Albuquerque news reporter, "but after we had that meeting, we just kept moving. It was clear we were committed."[27] By the end of the day, we had a plan that the staff supported.

We also had help from the community. As we struggled through those first days, friends from the Religious Coalition for Reproductive Choice came to bless us and feed us. Planned Parenthood agreed to let us use two of its clinics during available evenings and weekends when they weren't seeing their own patients. I turned to other clinics in Albuquerque where I had trained staff on counseling and where Curtis had filled in for their doctors in emergencies. Although we were competitors, in this larger battle, we were allies.

"It was like having your house burn down and having all your neighbors say, 'Come stay with us,'" Amanda told the local press. "We all felt a huge gratitude."

We were grateful, but it was hard on everyone as the weeks turned into months. After the Dallas arson, a frantic week of remediation was followed by a triumphant return to our familiar workplace, but the search for a replacement facility in Albuquerque stretched on indefinitely. Following such a dramatic attack, we couldn't find a medical facility that was willing to lease or sell to us. Many supported our work, but they did not want our troubles. We couldn't blame them.

We tried to find some humor in the situation. I invited staff to spill stories to me, and we took cold comfort in laughing as we cried. Two of our nurses would load their pickup trucks each morning with the supplies we'd need—sterile packs sealed in large plastic bins crammed against the portable suction machines and our precious sonogram machines, all wrapped and wedged in place with blankets. They drove with fingers crossed, hoping that nothing would break or fly out when they hit a speed bump. Our ultrasound tech was examining patients on an upholstered reclining chair in a Planned Parenthood doctor's cubicle—still private but hardly our usual standard of dignified medical care. The amazing thing is that patients never complained. Indeed, they were grateful.

Whenever work has been especially demanding, Curtis has invoked the image of swans, serene and elegant, gliding gracefully across the water while paddling like hell beneath. In those difficult months, we were swans. As a result, every patient scheduled in *The Book* received her abortion.

One of those patients brought us important news.

As Molly started to give her the preoperative IV medications, the patient looked into her eyes and said, "I think I know who burned your clinic."

As we performed her abortion, she told Molly her story. Stuck in an abusive relationship, she had learned she was pregnant and knew she had to get out. Such stories are not uncommon among women deciding to abort a pregnancy: realizing that they would never subject a child to the abuse they have tolerated, they gather the courage to leave—to finally protect themselves. When this young woman had told the ex-boyfriend that she was pregnant and planned to have an abortion, he'd become (as she later told the arson investigators) extremely upset.

The pieces of this puzzle soon fell into place. Joan remembered an agitated young man in a trench coat pacing in our waiting room the day before the arson. He'd come to the reception window repeatedly, asking odd questions and trying to peer into the secure clinic space separated from our waiting room by a locked door. Joan had kept an eye on him. He'd made her uneasy. Now she knew why.

The patient's disclosure coincided with a tip from the man's room-mate, which led to the speedy arrest of two men—both in their early twenties, drug addicted, and with no affiliation to any anti-abortion groups. Virtually all abortion facility arsons and bombings are perpe-trated by members of anti-abortion groups. They are organized, stra-tegically timed—Christmas, New Year's, and the Fourth of July are fa-vored dates—and the perpetrators are seldom caught. Sergio Baca and his friend Chad Altman were not terrorists acting in the service of a religious or political agenda. This was domestic violence gone public.

For years, Curtis has told our friends about one of our regular pick-eters in Dallas—a middle-aged man who carried the same handmade sign every day for years: *What Man Would Allow His Baby to Be Aborted?* Again and again, Curtis is baffled when his male friends don't see why that placard is so offensive. "What's wrong with that?" they say. "If I had a girlfriend who was pregnant, I'd care."

"That man is saying the pregnancy is *his property*," Curtis patiently explains. "He's saying that as long as his baby is in her uterus, *she* is his property too. She has no rights—no say in the decision." Curtis grew up in that kind of patriarchal world. Our arsonists personified that world-view. It's the world we hoped—and still hope—to change.

With perfect irony, the case came to trial as we were finally mov-ing into our new facility. We had been patching together patient care in

Albuquerque for nearly a year, traveling between several borrowed sites. It had been a long, emotional roller coaster for our staff. Once again, though, the community was behind us: Our realtor had found the right building. Friends who knew the owner had interceded on our behalf. And our banker fought with her institution for our mortgage. It was, as always, a team effort, but we managed to buy the place.

. . . .

The federal prosecutor met with us in our new office. We had a choice to make: Baca and Altman could be charged under federal law, which carried a sentence of up to twenty years in prison. Or they could be charged under state law, which meant they could be free in less than five years. How did we want to proceed?

We never discussed the decision, making our choice without a second thought. Curtis remembered lines from the Lord's Prayer: *Forgive us our trespasses, as we forgive those who trespass against us.* I heard my mother's stern voice when I was tempted to act spitefully: *Two wrongs don't make a right.* From our very different backgrounds, we were of one mind. We knew that twenty years in prison would restore neither our clinic nor our treasured illusion of safety in the world, but it could surely ruin the lives of those two troubled men. Against the wishes of many of our staff, we opted for the lesser penalty. They were charged at the state, not the federal, level.

Sergio Baca and Chad Altman pled guilty in federal court on January 7, 2009. For our safety, the federal officials asked us not to attend the trial, but many of our staff were present for the sentencing. So were most of the forty firefighters who had risked their lives on that December night thirteen months earlier. At the sentencing, Joan spoke for herself and for all of us by recounting the disruption to her life and the lives of all our staff—not just professionally, but personally. She concluded by saying, "I want you to know in your hearts and feel in your minds that you did a terribly wrong crime. I want the crime punished appropriately.

I want the world to know that we, as a society, do not allow this crime."[28] The two convicts apologized to Joan, and the firefighters thanked her for speaking for them, and from her heart.

Both men were out of prison in three years. We would like to believe that their experience changed them for the better—clean and sober would be a good start. As always, Curtis is more optimistic than I am about their chances. But I cling to the knowledge that our patient got out of an abusive relationship and the hope that she moved forward in her life.

It was time for us to move on with ours.

· · · ·

Anti-abortion harassment and violence have been an undeniable reality in our lives since the first United States clinic arson in 1975. When attacks increased in the 1980s, Curtis and I had long personal conversations about our own safety and how best to protect our patients and staff. We sought advice from several security firms and implemented many of their recommendations, but we did not want to turn our warm and welcoming clinics into armed fortresses. We would not—in truth, we could not—live in fear.

We had to accept that there are always risks and we cannot control all of them. Abiding by our decision is an act of will guided by a basic principle of mindfulness: we give the object of our focus power in our lives. Curtis and I refuse to give anti-abortion violence that power by focusing on it. That said, we do not live in denial of facts, and the statistics on anti-abortion violence are telling.

The National Abortion Federation began tracking violence and disruption at abortion facilities across North America in 1977, at a time of relative tranquility. The data, available on the NAF website, establish several trends.[29] First, there has been an exponential increase in all anti-abortion violence from 1977 to the present. In the early years of legal abortion (1977 through 1989), NAF tallied just over two thousand incidents of violence and disruption, while this past decade (2010 through 2019) witnessed over half a million such incidents. Even more disturbing, as the destruction of property continued during the 1990s, the violence escalated to murder.

Naturally, our worst fears shifted to the murders. Doctors, staff, volunteer escorts, security guards, and police officers at abortion clinics across the nation were killed. Since 1991 there have been eleven murders and another twenty-six attempted murders.[30]

The needs—not to mention the health and safety—of pregnant women got lost in the story of a "holy war." This change had a chilling effect on abortion providers and a numbing effect on the American public. For most Americans, such incidents became old news: *Another clinic arson? Another doctor shot?* For us, they became part of daily life.

Our clinic logbooks from both Dallas and Albuquerque are filled with weekly, even daily, accounts of taunts and threats against patients and staff—of shattered windows, broken doors, slashed car tires, and clinic blockades. We endured several clinic invasions, with protesters assaulting staff and chaining themselves to our equipment, forcing us to install automatic locks on every door. Curtis and I have both been stalked, as have staff and their family members—including their young children. We've had death threats hand-delivered to the front door of our home and our doctors' homes. The additional security measures we have taken are essential, but they do not guarantee safety.

That has not stopped us from carrying on our work.

While we grappled with the legal and criminal challenges, colleagues across the nation were similarly besieged. Most notably, our friend George Tiller was under attack.

Our friendship with George grew each time we met and on phone calls between meetings, especially after his visit to Dallas in the early 1980s. He was unfailingly caring toward us and honest about his own professional, as well as some personal, joys and struggles.

Curtis and George had many things in common, from their quiet dignity to their zany enthusiasm—especially for their children and grandchildren.

George grew up in a relatively affluent family in Wichita, Kansas, a much larger community than Curtis's hometown, although it was equally conservative. His father was a highly regarded physician who helped found the state's first residency program in family medicine—then a new specialty. When George completed his medical training with an internship in the US Navy, followed by training as a flight surgeon, he planned to begin a residency in dermatology. In 1970, however, his parents, sister, and brother-in-law were killed when the private plane piloted by his father, Jack, crashed. George and his wife, Jeanne, returned to Wichita with their firstborn baby in tow to adopt their one-year-old nephew—determined that he would never be treated as an orphan but as their son—and to carry on Jack's thriving general practice.

As Jeanne later explained to me, George came home from a long day's work one day in early 1973 with a story: "I have patients asking me to take care of them the way my father did. They're pregnant, and they need an abortion."[31] Abortion was newly legal, and George told Jeanne that, although surprised, he wasn't really shocked by the revelation that Jack—a pillar of the Kansas medical community—had quietly performed illegal abortions for the families in his care. "It was the sort of thing Dad would have done," George told Jeanne. "It was the right thing to do . . . and it still is." George was already committed to women's equal rights, and providing abortions at Women's Health Care Services became another unplanned legacy that he would openly and proudly carry on.

This parallel with Curtis's life is still striking to me. It wasn't until 1989 (twenty-two years after he performed his first abortion for Sallie) that Curtis learned his beloved grandmother, too, had provided abortions for her community. That was sixteen years after Mama Boyd—midwife, abortionist, and devout foot-washing Baptist—had died. While her work had no direct influence on Curtis's decision to perform abortions, this coincidental similarity with George's life story has prompted us to wonder: How many devoted doctors across America had quietly, secretly, provided illegal abortions, despite the dangers—compelled to act out of compassion for patients they knew and cared for? We will never know the answer to that question.

Although both George and Curtis were raised in deeply religious, conservative communities, George remained a part of his hometown community and faithful to his Christian roots. Many Sundays he served as an usher at the Reformation Lutheran Church, greeting parishioners old and new, while Jeanne sang in the church choir. She worried about George's exposure to strangers, but he was irrepressibly friendly. Plus, he had worn body armor under his clothes since 1988, when the FBI warned him that he was the target of anti-abortion extremist groups.

Jeanne had good reason to worry. In 1993, George was shot in both arms as he drove into his clinic parking lot, hunted down by a self-proclaimed anti-abortion terrorist, Rachelle Shannon. He returned to his clinic the following day to support his staff and the doctors who worked with him, and soon returned to performing abortions—even before his arms were fully healed.

George was truly irrepressible. A decade after that shooting, he created T-shirts for the NAF Annual Meeting. On the front, beneath the slogan *We Can Do It* and above the words *Team Tiller*, the familiar image of Rosie the Riveter smiled, her arm flexed in a gesture of female strength. On the back he added *Reproductive Ministry to Women* to his clinic logo. If only I still had that T-shirt!

George never lost his sense of humor, and his commitment to serving women never wavered. He was one of the few doctors to perform abortions in the third trimester of pregnancy, thus providing a safety net for patients whose pregnancies were untenable but beyond our gestational limit. Women came from all over the United States and the world to see him. He neither passed judgment nor questioned a woman's motives. His motto was simple and encompassing: *Trust women.* Between friends he also said, "Keep the faith."

Then on May 31, 2009—Memorial Day—George Tiller was assassinated in his church.

That Sunday morning, George was serving as an usher, greeting the faithful in the church foyer. As he extended his hand in welcome to a parishioner, a stranger, Scott Roeder, pointed a gun at George's head and fired at point-blank range.

Dr. George Tiller's assassination was devastating. We loved him. George did not become a hero in death—he enjoyed that status in his lifetime, with us and with so many abortion providers and activists. Our home phone rang constantly upon the news of his murder as our staff and colleagues from all over the country called to grieve with us. We needed to hear each other's voices, to cry together, and to ask aloud: "What will become of late-term abortion? Where will we send the desperate patients we cannot serve?"

Curtis and I imagined the answer, in part. George had trained two women doctors who became unemployed when his death forced Women's Health Care Services to close. The solution seemed simple: We would invite doctors Susan Robinson and Shelley Sella to practice in our clinic in Albuquerque. We would officially expand our gestational limit and let the abortion-providing community know that George's work would continue in New Mexico.

Like many simple solutions, the reality proved more complicated. It held some surprises too.

. . . .

We had seen our "simple solution" while we were still in shock over George's murder, thinking, *Of course, we must do this, and we will make it work.* Before we even made a move, Dr. Robinson called Curtis about the possibility of working for us. She and Dr. Sella were looking out for each other and wanted to job-share as they had with George. This attitude of mutual support suggested they could be a good fit with our team approach to the work. We talked it over with our staff and then invited the doctors to visit our clinic in Albuquerque, meet the staff, and assess the prospect as realistically as possible.

The meeting with our staff was essential, allowing them to ask questions and voice their concerns openly. Among our staff, we talk with ease about the importance of patients being at peace with their abortion. Although we seldom speak of it publicly, Curtis and I have that same concern for ourselves and our staff. An abortion is a brief event in a patient's life, so it seldom becomes central to their sense of themselves. But for those of us who choose this work, it becomes part of our identity, often a significant part. Our staff need to feel a level of comfort with the procedure and a deep appreciation of its complex, nuanced meaning—not only in the lives of our patients, but in their own lives.

To a person, the staff recognized the need and supported the idea of moving forward with third-trimester abortions. Their commitment to abortion as a fundamental right was absolute, and most foresaw no problem in expanding our gestational limit. Only two staff members disclosed their doubts about being able to deal emotionally with larger, more developed pregnancies. Their reservations were grounded in their personal lives: a premature birth saved by heroic measures for one, and the heartbreak of stillbirth for the other—each within the gestational limits we would now be seeing. I appreciated their honesty.

In the fall of 2009, Dr. Robinson and Dr. Sella joined our Albuquerque staff, and we all learned new skills and faced new challenges—together. The more difficult abortions they had learned to perform carry a risk of serious complications equivalent to the risk in full-term deliveries; bleeding and infection remain the most common. However, the risks of uterine rupture of a previous C-section scar and DIC (the rare complication that took Angela's life) are also greater—as they are with childbirth. Realistically, both patients and staff are committing to a longer, more physically demanding process with a greater risk of serious complications.

We remodeled portions of our building to create spaces tailored to the needs of these new patients, and we adapted to the wave of patients who came to us from all parts of the United States and Canada.

The leaders of the anti-abortion group that had harassed George and his staff for years—and, significantly, had been in phone contact with his assassin on the day of George's murder—adapted too. They moved from Wichita to Albuquerque. The couple parked what George had called their "trash truck" in front of our clinic. The midsize moving van, with its exterior walls and rear door covered in blown-up stock photos of bloody body parts (that may or may not have been from aborted fetuses), also served as their mobile home. Daily harassment of our patients and staff intensified. Yet again, we increased our security measures.

I spoke privately with the two staff members who had expressed doubts and agreed that to determine what they could and could not handle, we would learn by doing. Both were experienced, committed to our philosophy of patient care, and cross-trained to fill several roles. As things unfolded, both of them stayed with us for their entire career—one working closely with the third-trimester patients, and the other learning new office skills.

Several staff who had previously expressed no qualms about third-trimester abortion did leave our clinic within the year but remained committed to abortion rights. One completed her PhD in anthropology and got the university professorship of her dreams. The other two found the reality of these medically induced miscarriages more demanding than they had imagined. These late-term procedures take longer—usually three days but occasionally four—and often require night work. The process is more painful for patients, and witnessing pain is also hard on the staff, as we had learned when developing our second-trimester program.

We had been so grateful to refer these challenging cases to George, knowing that they would be managed with skill and compassion. Although the number of abortions performed in the third trimester is minuscule—a fraction of the one percent of patients served after twenty-four weeks—they are among the most desperately needed. When catastrophic threats to the life and health of the pregnancy or the woman emerge as the pregnancy progresses, the woman and her family are often devastated. When third-trimester patients' lives are further complicated by poverty, homelessness, physical abuse, or drug addiction—with the risks to life and health inherent in those social ills—the situation is undeniably desperate. The raw sorrow in all these situations makes the work demanding, but for staff who thrive on challenge, it is also particularly rewarding.

Doctors Sella and Robinson deserve praise for continuing this important work, and we are glad that we could provide a home for them.

Both doctors have since retired. The Tiller family carries on George's legacy through a family foundation, the George R. Tiller, MD, Memorial Fund for the Advancement of Women's Health.[32] I wish George was alive to write his story in his own words, but Jeanne says that whenever she urged him to slow down and write about his experiences, his answer was clear: "My story will be told in the lives of the women I helped."

. . . .

All these hard times and disturbing experiences have challenged Curtis and me, but over time the pain fades. Meanwhile, the ways we are changed endure. For reasons I will probably never understand, Curtis and I share a determination to emerge from hard times with our trust in the world and our goodwill toward others intact, hoping to become better people—and wiser for our troubles.

Our goal now is to continue training gifted physicians so women continue to have options throughout their pregnancies. However, we carry on this important work with hard-earned caution. The predictable medical complications with the third trimester have occurred and, tragically, a second patient death from DIC in 2017. In contrast to the relative media calm around Angela's death in 1980, this one was broadcast far and wide by anti-abortion websites. An anti-abortion attorney persuaded the patient's mother to sue us, and that suit attracted further adverse attention—all of which occurred as the video falsely portraying Planned Parenthood as "selling aborted baby parts for profit" was making another round in the national news.

Planned Parenthood was not selling fetal tissue, but that story did reveal something shocking: we were now living in a post-fact world. Anti-abortion legislators in the US House of Representatives convened the Select Investigative Panel on Infant Lives in response to the faked videos and focused on our work for a time. The personal and professional assault we had feared so many years earlier with Angela's death did materialize in the end, and the emotional toll on our doctors and staff was—and still is—greater than I can calculate. As the statistics on anti-abortion harassment and violence make clear, the social and political environment is far more hostile in tone and violent in action than it was fifty years ago.

We were also changed.

Angela's death occurred when both of my parents were still alive, when I had not yet had cancer—when my original world was largely intact. The tragedy of her death was a first for me. As I sat on that bench in the Dallas surgery area waiting for the bad news from Parkland Hospital, I realized that I had turned a corner in life. Something important—life-and-death important—was happening, and I had no control. Angela would die, and my life would never be the same. I did not know what would come, only that I was not in control.

Thirty-seven years later, Curtis and I were not present for the second death. We were at work in Dallas when we got the call. I wanted to scream *No!* to the universe. Instead, we went into action, gathering the facts of the case and traveling to Albuquerque to be with our staff.

The patient, a young and healthy woman named Rose, had been in the preparatory stage of the abortion, with osmotic dilators in her cervix and on medication to stimulate uterine contractions. Our doctor, Shawna Carter, sensed that something was wrong: the patient's oxygen level had dropped, with no apparent cause.[33] Dr. Carter put Rose on supplemental oxygen, and the staff monitored her closely, but her oxygen level remained unexplainably low.

In line with the protocol we'd developed following Angela's death, Dr. Carter called for an ambulance to transfer Rose to the university hospital for observation and ongoing management. It seemed an unnecessary precaution, but something wasn't right, and our guiding principle is to err on the side of patient safety.

By the time Rose arrived at the hospital ER, she looked worse to Dr. Carter, who met the ER team. She was in respiratory distress and went into sudden cardiac arrest about seven hours later. After heroic attempts to resuscitate her failed, Rose was declared dead. That's when we got the call.

It was pure heartache. Rose's cardiac arrest did not occur on our exam table, but otherwise the pattern was so similar to our experience with Angela. For Curtis, once again, there was no medical puzzle to solve, no new protocols to develop. The medical examiner determined that the immediate cause of death had been a pulmonary embolus—a complication of pregnancy, not abortion—which triggered the cascade of events that led to fatal DIC. But in the politically charged atmosphere of 2017, the facts were ignored.

As I tried to comfort staff, it became a deeper lesson in accepting what I could not control, not only the patient's death and the media attention but how others—a new generation of doctors and staff—manage their sense of loss and grief. Within the clinic, we grieved, each in our own way and collectively, but our grief was highjacked by hostile assaults from the media and protesters.

"Unless you've lived it, no one understands what a maternal death feels like," Dr. Carter shared with me years later. "Deaths are so rare with abortion. We have to report these events, and the one in 2017, it was me."[34] Not *mine*, but *me*—as if a part of her died with that experience.

As an OB-GYN with years of experience, Dr. Carter had never experienced a patient death even though they're more common in general obstetrical practice than in the abortion setting. Six years later, she said, "A patient death never leaves you. I still see her beautiful face. She was so young." Dr. Carter recognized the importance of talking about these things and being honest about the pain, both as a way to honor the patient and to care for herself. Like Dr. Carter, Curtis and I have faith that even tragedy can offer opportunities for deep reflection and valuable personal growth.

On some level, Dr. Carter pointed out, we're always having a conversation about life and death—not only the risk to the patient but the life and death of her pregnancy: "The patient knows what she is doing, and I know what I'm doing, and sometimes it is painful. . . . When we share that pain, I want the patient to know that she is not alone. I don't know how to put in words how special that is. This work is a privilege."

Part III

Our Philosophy

CHAPTER NINE

Stories: Learning from Our Patients

*"Tolerance and being non-judgmental are beautiful things.
You never know what someone is dealing with until you
experience it for yourself. PRO-CHOICE!!!:-)"*
—*Patient journal entry*

Glenna

When I agreed to train the first generation of legal abortion counselors in the US Southwest, the field did not exist, and anyway, my qualifications were laughable. I was both a feminist and an atheist with my own history and ties to each of those groups. In truth, everything I know about abortion counseling, I learned from patients.

Even in those early days of legal abortion, I had known that I'd have to develop my own approach to abortion counseling. As with most important things in my life, I underestimated the scope of the task. With women's right to abortion secured, I assumed that my previous work with difficult social issues had prepared me for this much easier job: I would be done with abortion counseling in about six months and then move on. Instead, I've spent most of my career as a witness to the soul-searching work of women, couples, and families as they decide whether to continue or end a pregnancy. I had no idea that their soul-searching would require a corresponding search on my part.

My experiences with our patients quickly set me straight.

The existing traditions informing the abortion counselor's approach were grounded in doctrine: either feminism or religion. As a feminist, I wanted to hear and respect each woman's unique experience. Although I personally rejected the clergy's casting of abortion as a sin and the "lesser of evils," our patients were teaching me to respect religious and moral concerns. Yet I wanted to anchor abortion counseling instead in something else: women's experience.

From day one, a single principle had hit me in the face, and it guides our abortion counseling to this day: *The patient's feelings, beliefs, and needs are paramount.* Our task—for anyone who works with patients, not only designated counselors—is to create a safe place for patients to voice them.

Early in my career, a young patient caught me by surprise, sharing more complex thinking and deeper feelings than I expected or was prepared to hear. Emily was an eighteen-year-old mother with a two-year-old and a newborn. She had dropped out of high school during her first pregnancy because motherhood was her dream come true. Now her two children were the center of her life, but she and her husband struggled to support them. This pregnancy occurred while she was breastfeeding, despite her doctor's assurance that would not happen, and she didn't have the physical or emotional strength to have another baby so soon. She and her husband had talked it over again and again, spending sleepless nights, knowing they just couldn't make it work.

Emily was articulate, emotional, and clear-headed. She knew what needed to be done and was prepared to do it with the full support of her husband. As she talked, she opened her wallet to show me a photo of her two children snuggled in her arms. Resting her free hand on her newly pregnant belly, she said, "This is my third child. I have to sacrifice him or her. I know what I'm doing, and it breaks my heart."

I was the one choking back tears. The photo of Emily with her two beloved children hit a nerve.

Women know what they are doing. They don't need a counselor, a sonogram, a clergyman, or the state to tell them that the pregnancy they carry will develop into a baby. The majority of women having abortions in the United States today already have one or more children.[35] They know the demands of motherhood, and they are better equipped than anyone else to make the decision that they will have to live with.

However, Emily taught me a more personal lesson. I had never needed an abortion myself, so my understanding was intellectual, not visceral. With her tenth-grade education, Emily thought and felt more fully and honestly about her conflicting feelings than I had allowed myself to feel about the work I was coming to love. She could simultaneously hold the belief that this pregnancy was her third child *and* assume responsibility for ending it. If she could act with sadness and love, but without shame or guilt, then perhaps I could help others along that journey.

I had work to do.

. . . .

I needed to develop a counseling protocol that would translate my intuitive approach into topics and questions that all counselors could use as their guide, and I hoped the historical record could be of help. Abortion has existed throughout all recorded history and in every known culture, yet undoubtedly the history of abortion is so long as to predate written record. In 1955, French anthropologist Georges Devereaux characterized abortion as one of the "problems which have beset mankind since the dawn of time . . . which man can neither ignore, nor resolve, nor learn to live with."[36] In that regard, sadly, he may have been prescient.

As Devereaux documented, abortion—like much of women's experience—was shrouded in secrecy and silence. Its implementation varied from closely held secret knowledge to open but unspoken practice, usually by women's clans or societies. In the United States, abortion was routinely performed by lay midwives until the late 1800s, when the emerging profession of medicine claimed pregnancy management as part of its domain. Nascent medical organizations began to promote legislation to regulate abortion, or even make it illegal, out of self-interest—to exclude amateurs from the practice of medicine.

Staking their claim to the care of pregnant women required eliminating the competition, but these physician groups also had genuine concerns for women's health and safety. Death in childbirth was not uncommon, and home remedies to end untimely pregnancies were both dangerous and often ineffective. The newly formed medical societies seldom expressed religious or moral objections to ending a pregnancy, and although abortion was redefined as a medical issue, not a women's issue, midwives and others continued to perform abortions much as they always had. Taking care of things on their own terms, after all, is at the core of women's experience.

I know this from personal experience. As a novice counselor, I would occasionally field an urgent phone call from a woman in South Dallas who had been doing abortions in her neighborhood for years. My work with the Dallas Urban League had shown me just how racially segregated Dallas was, so the fact that she lived and worked in South Dallas told me that she was undoubtedly a Black woman with a loyal following, and even after legalization, the people of her community continued to see her rather than travel across the river to White Dallas and our legal abortion clinic. She must have known through the grapevine that Curtis had performed illegal abortions too, and that's why she trusted him, occasionally making an urgent phone call: "I got a trouble, and I need the good doctor's help."

Curtis took her calls promptly and talked her through the problem, treating her as he would any medical colleague—sometimes prescribing an antibiotic or asking whether someone could drive the patient to our clinic so he could safely complete the abortion. He made no secret of this practice; these patients came and left through our front door. Their care was expedited, they were never charged, and no record was made. At the time, I had no idea of the medical and legal risks he was taking, but his kindness and pragmatic acceptance of this earnest lay-midwife and her patients was among the acts that endeared him to me—then and to this day.

Abortion has been practiced forever and probably always will be, regardless of medical organizations or fanatic terrorists or disingenuous regulations. Yet I found no evidence in previous eras that anything resembling counseling accompanied the act. The actual history of abortion counseling is short, spanning less than seventy years in the United States. Even so, I had to sort through previous traditions, not dismiss them. I had to examine my own philosophical biases so I didn't unwittingly impose them on patients or staff.

I took another, deeper look at what I knew about the prevailing doctrines. Curtis's allies in the Clergy Consultation Service were the first in the United States to begin exploring the potential of counseling, in the 1960s. Many Protestant denominations wrote formal position papers in support of abortion rights, recognizing women's need for abortion and the wisdom of making it safe and legal. Simultaneously, the emerging feminist movement was lobbying and testifying for legal abortion while also promoting self-abortion and teaching women to perform "menstrual extractions" for each other—a practice that was sometimes simply a means of getting through menstruation quickly but sometimes a euphemism for terminating an extremely early pregnancy. Both traditions held a common, deep value: Women must have control over their own bodies.

Despite their work to legalize abortion and thus forever change the place of women in American society, both the clergy and the feminists had deep ties to the ways of the past—the CCS as open-minded, compassionate members of their faith traditions, and the feminists as an outspoken version of the far older tradition of closed women's societies. Consequently, these two social movements approached the question of how to help women deal with the decision in very different ways.

The CCS members, who were virtually all men, saw their role as twofold: to protect the doctors of conscience they had recruited to do prelegal abortions, and to ensure that women obtaining abortions could live with their decision. They intended the single-page "Guide to Counseling in Problem Pregnancy" to help their clergy protect women from regret and guilt, earnest in their wish that each woman determine which decision best met her needs in the context of her religious or moral beliefs and her life situation. Admittedly, there was a paternalistic element in the assumption that women in distress need guidance in making their determination. However, my experience suggested that most patients welcome a sympathetic ear and reassurance that their thoughts and feelings are understood. Major life decisions provoke anxiety and are, by their nature, isolating. We all benefit from hearing ourselves talk out loud to a caring listener.

In contrast, the official feminist position of the time was that abortion was simply a woman's right. The politically correct feminist approach bypassed the woman's decision-making process: her reasoning and feelings were no one's business. To counsel abortion seekers smacked of resurrecting the "special exemptions" standard of prelegal days, when well-connected women could obtain abortions in many non-Catholic hospitals in the United States. Rape, incest, and threat to the life of the mother were commonly accepted reasons to end a pregnancy. As states liberalized their abortion laws prior to 1973, many states added "psychiatric indications" to the list. If a woman was judged by the designated medical authority as suicidal or otherwise "unfit," she could obtain an abortion. From the feminist perspective, prior to 1973 the men's club of medicine had ruled, and counseling women prior to an abortion merely perpetuated that injustice.

The FWHC was ambivalent about, if not hostile to, the medicalization of abortion. Its nonphysician staff, designated as patient advocates, provided a factual description of the procedure to patients in groups to speed their care. The FWHC wanted to keep the cost of abortion low, get the procedure over with quickly, and discourage any displays of emotion. This philosophy bordered on a macho ethic: "Real women" were not emotional about their decision. Women could and would take care of themselves and each other. I appreciated the history that guided the feminist position but believed this version of counseling denied patients free expression of their feelings and, in assuming the role of patient advocate, unintentionally disempowered the actual patients—in direct conflict with feminist ideology, which holds that women advocate for themselves and be heard in their own voices.

As my experiences with patients forced me to reconsider my initial rejection of the two approaches, I came to appreciate the good intentions and wisdom in both the feminist and the clergy perspectives, discovering that I could make use of both while conforming to neither.

One of the most significant health care contributions of the feminist movement was their emphasis on education and fully informed consent. I already recognized patient education as a part of counseling—but not the whole. Our consent forms from 1973 forward have listed the true known risks, providing detailed descriptions as well as their rates of occurrence—all of which was often far more than patients wanted to know. Of course, abortion patients want safety. But like most of us facing a medical procedure, they seldom want to dwell on the risks. As I carefully explained each risk, their eyes would glaze over. Most would just pick up the pen and say, "Show me where to sign."

When a patient *is* focused on the risks, there is always a story behind that fear, and I learned to elicit the story. Offering statistical reassurance rings hollow; taking patients' fears seriously can give us useful information as well as the opportunity to make clear that we want to avoid problems too—that we are as invested in our patients' safety as they are.

Given our focus on safety, and the underlying feminist history behind fully informed consent, it is ironic that much of the state-by-state anti-abortion legislation in the 1990s and since has been based on the claim that women are not "told the truth about the grave dangers of abortion." A first-trimester abortion is one of the safest medical procedures in the United States, so it is a cruel paradox that this legislation—justified as "necessary" for women's health and safety—mandates a campaign of disinformation about risks, suggesting that abortion directly causes breast cancer or infertility.

If my commitment to informed consent was aligned with the feminists, I took something more complicated from the CCS approach. Years of honing our counseling approach helped me recognize the symbolic power of being referred for an abortion by a minister. In such cases, whatever a woman's religious or spiritual inclinations, she knows that her abortion is accepted by an agent of God. Although the symbolism was initially lost on me, the importance of religion to many patients came through loud and clear as patients told me their stories.

To center the patient's experience, I settled on a simple, direct question: *What religious or spiritual beliefs do you hold that might affect how you're feeling about this abortion?* It's a question with no right answer. Only the woman's point of view—and perhaps that of her partner or family—matters. The tone of voice and body language accompanying the patient's reply determine where the counseling goes from there.

To this day, I use that same direct question in counseling sessions. It lends dignity to thoughts and feelings patients may lack the words to express, and it helps us both understand the significance of the abortion—not to me or anyone else but to the individual woman.

. . . .

Curtis knew from his early experience that counseling made a difference. Patients referred through the CCS were calmer and more trusting, and they had far less pain with the procedure. Like most physicians then and now, however, Curtis was trained to focus on physical care, to diagnose and treat illness and injury: take charge, solve problems, prescribe medications, give advice, perform surgery. Beyond that, until I showed up with a more concerted focus on "attending to the emotional needs of patients" (as he put it), Curtis relied on his natural kindness and good manners.

I, too, brought my own personality and experiences to the philosophy and practice we developed. For one, I started from the assumption that a crisis intervention model would be most fitting for a one-time counseling encounter with women I assumed were in the midst of a life crisis—and I was so wrong.

Patients taught me that the abortion was seldom a crisis. The *pregnancy* is the crisis; abortion is the resolution of that crisis. The most common emotion patients express after the abortion is relief.

I was also confident that meaningful abortion counseling needed to be done individually, which probably reflects my own private nature.

I would never discuss my feelings, beliefs, or internal conflicts with a group of strangers.

In individual private sessions, I learned to listen carefully to the issues patients raised, searching for common threads while also reflecting on the psychological theories that could guide my own thinking and offer perspective and comfort to patients. To guide and clarify my own thinking, I made a list of the things patients commonly talked about. I called it "The Tendrils of Abortion." A nod to my youth in California wine country, the mental image of grape vines sending out intertwining shoots for additional support as they grow was intended to honor the connection many women feel to the pregnancy and to recognize the ties that abortion has to innumerable aspects of a woman's life. I wanted to help the entire staff see each pregnancy, and the decision to continue or end it, in the context of the patient's life—to appreciate the unique meaning abortion holds for her.

My approach was direct: *Tell me what is going on in your life that brought you to us to end your pregnancy.* Guided by patients' storytelling over time, I developed a list of six key areas that often call out for our attention:

1. Beliefs and feelings about pregnancy in general: hopes, dreams, and fears
2. The meaning of this pregnancy in particular
3. Beliefs about abortion in general and feelings about this abortion in particular
4. The impact of this pregnancy and abortion on important relationships—the man, parents, whomever, including god
5. Hopes for future childbearing
6. Thoughts or plans for birth control in the future, including ways we could help with contraception

Those six points became a mental checklist for the counselor to hold in mind as the patient tells her story. With this list of relevant topics clear in my own mind, I am free to listen without fear of getting lost in patients' wandering stories. Following the patient's train of thought instead of a preset list of questions also keeps the counseling, which could become boringly routine, alive and real for staff as well as patients.

I am regularly struck by how relieved, even grateful, patients are to share intimate details of their lives when they realize we are actively listening. When patients feel safe with us, most will raise some or all of these issues even without prompting. If they do not mention an issue, the counselor can then use her judgment in raising that topic or not. Having children someday may be irrelevant to a twelve-year-old rape victim. On the other hand, a thirty-five-year-old woman aborting her first pregnancy may be relieved to learn that prospects for future childbearing are a frequent worry for women her age. That simple statement of fact does not force her to discuss the issue with us but may give her permission to explore a crucial implication of this abortion with us or with other significant people in her life.

Despite the importance of these "tendrils," I learned to stress with each patient that she is under no obligation to explain nor justify her decision. Counseling is never a test that the patient must pass in order to have an abortion. However, we do have an ethical and legal responsibility to determine that she is clear in her decision and that—although she is probably taking the needs and feelings of others into consideration—she is not being coerced in her decision. At the heart of counseling is an ethical responsibility to understand enough about a patient's emotional state for our doctor and counselor to sign her informed consent for treatment in good faith, confident that she is at peace with her decision or can come to a genuine acceptance of her actions. In short, we need to believe that by providing the abortion, we are doing her no harm.

For almost all patients, the decision to end a pregnancy is a significant one, and they treat it as such, taking time to weigh their options and talk with the most important people in their lives. But for most, the decision is not tortured. They feel confident they are doing the best thing, usually for everyone concerned, and they are ready to move on with their lives. For a few women, the decision is fraught. No matter what they do, loss and heartache, even danger, seem inevitable.

As the CCS's "Guide to Counseling in Problem Pregnancy" so powerfully explained, sometimes settling for the least bad option is the best we can do. Accepting that bitter truth—which occurs in many life situations—requires perspective, maturity, and the capacity to tolerate conflicting feelings. Together, we explore the patient's previous experience with loss and regret and reinforce existing coping skills. Honestly facing how hard her situation is, and making realistic predictions about how she will feel after the abortion, is necessary for both patients and staff. In rare cases, we recruit community resources beyond what we can offer; trusted psychotherapists and clergy are at the top of the list, but women's shelters and suicide prevention organizations have occasionally served as valuable resources. The most essential thing we can do while the patients are with us is let them know that they are not alone.

Our counselors strive to do one thing above all else: listen. Feeling heard is so rare in daily life, and yet it's nearly magical in its power to create a sense of human connection and, ultimately, to generate a sense of calm. Our willingness to see and hear our patients is especially urgent, both because we are strangers to them and because the controversy that hovers over abortion—the word, the act, the setting, and the people providing the service—adds layers of uncertainty and fear for most patients.

Whenever the decision to end a pregnancy is unusually difficult or conflicted, we form a plan for emotional coping and additional counseling after the abortion. Patients seem grateful for the offer of future support, yet they seldom call or return for further counseling.

In the early years, we included a post-op appointment in our routine of care.[37] *How have you been feeling since the procedure—physically and emotionally?* was the first question on the form the patient filled out as she waited to be examined by the nurse. The answers allowed the nurse to provide additional counseling when needed and, importantly, allowed me to help patients set more realistic expectations—not only for the varied patterns of cramping and bleeding but to normalize occasional weepy moments and the overwhelming sense of relief.

And I learned all of this the slow way: from experience, patient by patient.

. . . .

I have yet to meet a patient who *wants* an abortion. It's simply not on anyone's bucket list of life experiences. And yet the need is ever present. This conflict underscores the theory that came to guide our abortion counseling. And Emily—the wise young mother whose photo with her two children brought me to tears—pointed me to it.

Being a mother was the most important thing in her life, and she wanted a third child, but not now. Few patients arrive at the clinic with Emily's clarity and capacity to accept the gulf between what we want and what life sometimes gives us. She wanted not to be pregnant; she didn't want an abortion. And as she spoke with me, she could hold her wish for a third child and her decision to abort her third pregnancy in her hands simultaneously. Although she was torn, she was not torn apart . . . not from herself, from her husband, or from their children. Her identity and her family were intact.

Emily demonstrated a level of comfort with her ambivalence that taught me the power of owning our inner conflicts. It was as if she'd held a mirror up and I saw myself in the glass. Once my eyes were opened to the push and pull between competing needs and desires, I started to see it everywhere in my life, and I started to value the ability to tolerate conflicting hopes, dreams, and feelings—in myself and others. Few important life experiences are free from inner conflict. We are forced to make choices, and every big decision (and plenty of smaller ones) has gains and losses. The greater my capacity to feel these conflicts within myself, the more authentically I could meet each patient wherever she was with her abortion experience.

With this new perspective, I could ground my abortion counseling in a theoretical context: existentialism. Most abortion patients are anxious about more than the procedure. *Will I regret my decision? Will it define how others see me? How can I be sure?* In other words, what meaning will the abortion hold in their lives over time? Many of our patients are living an existential dilemma: struggling with choice, freedom, anxiety, and the search for meaning—all key concepts of the philosophy, and all central to the abortion experience. Choice and freedom in particular (catchwords of the cause in the 1960s and 70s) are sources of anxiety because we must take action without knowledge of outcomes, as existential philosophers from Soren Kierkegaard to Paul Tillich have noted.[38] The painful truth is, we all have to make major life decisions without a crystal ball. We all lie awake at night, worrying whether we're making the "right" decision.

The struggles of decision-making can go on within ourselves or be played out with others. With the abortion decision, the conflict is frequently played out within the family—particularly between teens and their parents, with each party certain their vision of the future is the right one.

Camilla was fourteen years old when she arrived at the clinic accompanied by her mother. She was silent, even sullen, when I called her from the waiting room. As we sat in the counseling room, she pulled her long brown hair across her face like a veil, denying eye contact. I decided to get straight to what I suspected was the problem, explaining that I was meeting with her one-on-one because the decision to continue or end this pregnancy was hers and hers alone. I would not, and could not by law, force her to do anything against her will.

Without changing her posture, she flatly stated, "I don't want an abortion. I want to have this baby."

"Then we won't be doing an abortion today." I remained silent for a very long minute. When Camilla made no response, I continued. "I know your mother is here with you. She's signed all the consent forms." I flipped through the extra pages of paperwork required by the State of Texas and said, "It looks like she's even filled out your medical history form, so I'm guessing she wants you to have the abortion."

That broke Camilla's silence. "She did it all. It's her idea, but I'm not gonna do it."

"Sounds like you have a different plan for your future and the baby's."

I never know if a sullen teen will open up to me. But I've learned that using their words, reflecting their point of view, is my best chance. Some teens don't have any plan beyond defiance of their parents' will, and those teens seldom trust me at first.

In Camilla's case, she had a plan, and once I'd shown genuine interest, she spilled it. Her boyfriend wanted her to have "his baby," and his parents were prepared to take her into their home. Her plan was detailed, and his parents had done the same for an older son's pregnant girlfriend.

I asked Camilla if she had shared this plan with her mother.

"She just says I'm throwing my life away," Camilla replied, "and she doesn't want to hear about it."

"Hmm . . . Are you and your mother usually at odds?"

"Only about Jason. She's never liked him. Says he'll amount to nothing just like his whole family and only drag me down." With these words, Camilla began to cry, and more of the story emerged. "Mom had me when she was fourteen, and now she thinks I'm making the same mistake. That my life will be as hard as hers was."

"Sounds like she really cares about you."

"She does. She just doesn't understand that I'm not her. It'll all be different for me."

I smiled ruefully. "That's what we all hope. That our story will turn out better." After a pause, and now making eye contact, I took a risk: "Does any part of you worry that she might be right?"

Camilla's reply was swift and decisive. "Absolutely not!"

"OK. Are you ready to tell her that we won't do an abortion for you?"

"I have to."

"Do you want my help, or do you want to do it yourself?" I offered.

"Would you?"

"Of course. It's part of my job."

"Talk to her first without me. Please." That word was far more than courtesy. It was a plea.

I had Camilla wait in an available exam room while I called her mother from the waiting room. As we sat in the counseling room, I explained the situation to Camilla's mother, Jean. "We cannot by law as well as medical ethics perform an abortion without the patient's consent, and Camilla refuses to have this abortion."

In tears, Jean said, "She's making the same mistake I made at her age. Jason's family lives in squalor, and I've worked so hard to give her a better life." Then she looked into my eyes. "Is she doomed to repeat my history?" she asked, as if I could answer such a question.

Part of me wanted to cry and tell her how many mothers of pregnant teens have asked me that same question. Instead, I said, "She's early in the pregnancy. Can you let her go to live with them for now? Let her experience the reality, not her fantasy. If she changes her mind, we'll be here . . . for her, and for you."

We stood and hugged each other. I wrote *No AB* on Camilla's chart and felt, for neither the first nor the last time, how limited my powers are in the lives of others.

Working with abortion patients has schooled me to be grateful for the decisions that are not mine to make. In Camilla's case, my sympathies were with the worried mother. But in fact, none of us know how a story will turn out. All I can do is bear witness as each patient finds her way to the decision that is right for her. I never saw Camilla again, and I'm not betting on happily ever after, but it's unfair to dismiss her youthful optimism.

· · · ·

Are teens different from our other patients? The answer is yes and no, and the biological basis for difference becomes clearer as scientists continue to learn more about the development of the human brain.

The general public assumes that the majority of abortion patients are teenagers, but our direct experience tells me this is not so. The majority of our patients are between seventeen and twenty-seven years old, mirroring the years of highest female fertility. However, the anti-abortion movement, politicians, and thus the media have long been focused on the younger patients.

The standard political talking point in opposition to laws requiring parental consent for abortions is the need to protect children from abusive parents. However, in our experience, teenagers, especially younger ones, need and want their parent or parents involved in the decision and in the abortion. The most common reason younger patients give for keeping the abortion a secret is that they don't want to disappoint the parents they love. When probed, they divulge the secret they really want to keep from their family: that they are sexually active.

With younger patients who don't want to involve their family members, I've learned to ask, "Have you kept other important secrets from them?" My intent is not to pry. If the pregnancy is the first secret, it's a big one. That deserves to be acknowledged as an important step in developing an independent identity. Teens are part child, part adult, and we want to support their development. In such cases, that may be pivotal to how we can best serve the patient.

The other common motivation for teenagers to avoid telling their family is the fact that their parents have problems of their own, and the teens want to protect their parents from another source of worry. In this case, it can be useful to inquire about other adults the patient could turn to for support if needed. I then try to discuss if and when she will tell her parents.

What is often lost in discussions of teen pregnancy is how seriously many take the responsibilities of motherhood. The wish to be a good mother is the primary motive for many, if not most, abortions—regardless of the patient's age. The single most common patient statement we hear in our clinic is some variation of "I want to be the best mother I can be, and I can't *be that right now*." The reasons are unique to each patient's story, but the core sentiment is the same.

· · · ·

I can remember only three patients who revealed no tender feelings about their situation—and those three women could not have been more different from each other.

The first was the drug addict who deliberately vomited on me when the physician refused to give her more IV medication. She cared about only one thing: getting drugs.

The second was an abused teen living in a family with multiple ongoing incestuous relationships, which she relished describing in vivid detail. We made no reaction to her tales and added our report to what the local police in her rural Texas county told us was a long list.

The third was an attorney who had a serious fetal defect in a planned pregnancy. When I introduced myself to her, saying that I was sorry to meet under these circumstances, she immediately dismissed my concern. She said she was fine and never wavered from that position. She and her equally stoic attorney husband expressed neither sadness nor regret. The abortion was simply necessary business.

Although I still vividly remember the three women who appeared indifferent to their abortion, I cannot count the number of women who say, "I never thought I would do this!" This runs decidedly counter to the stereotype of women who have abortions. In the myth, they are frivolous teenagers or seasoned sluts—and I have met many teenagers and several sex workers in nearly fifty years of abortion counseling. However, our patient population generally reflects a cross-section of American women in their reproductive years. They are "ordinary" women who find themselves pregnant. Deciding whether to continue or end the pregnancy forces them to examine their values, plans, hopes, and dreams. It's a significant life event, and they know it.

These women are forever changed. Their sense of themselves and of the complexity of life expands—it's not always comfortable, but the enlarged space leaves room for the unknown, unknowable future. It's a profound lesson that applies to life in general: none of us can predict what we will actually do until we are faced with the reality. We hold opinions, state positions, but we do not know until we are there.

Realizing this is both humbling and humanizing. Many people experience this expansion only occasionally in their lifetimes. Through our patients, however, we experience it almost every day.

· · · ·

Knowing the overriding importance of social support in all areas of life, it's embarrassing to remember that when I began in this work, my brand of feminism was rather rigid. It excluded anyone other than the pregnant woman from all aspects of the abortion experience—except for providing transportation. Indeed, patients and their families and friends tried to set me straight.

In the early days of our practice, we refused to speak with anyone other than the pregnant woman—beginning with our first telephone contact. If a parent or boyfriend called, we provided brief general information about abortion, but we refused to make an appointment until we believed we had spoken directly with the prospective patient. In truth, we were often less than cordial with anyone acting as an intermediary. Of course, this attitude was in direct conflict with our recognition that trust and mutual respect must begin from the word *hello*.

It took me longer to abandon my rigid ideology than I care to admit. I had to experience being a patient myself, in urgent need of orthopedic care from a painful knee injury. When Curtis called the doctor for me, it hit me: caring for patients *includes* caring for the people who care for those patients too. The scar I bear from that knee surgery is a daily reminder to appreciate family and friends who show up on behalf of our patients.

We still meet with the patient alone for an individual counseling session—*before* including family, partners, or friends—to confirm that she is not being coerced into an abortion. But we learned that when a patient asks to include someone important in the session, we should welcome that person. That is how I met both Linda and James.

Linda's medical history stated she was in her midthirties, a bit older than most of our patients. She reported five living children ranging in age from seventeen to three. She had experienced one miscarriage and reported no previous abortions. Our ultrasound revealed that she was in her eighteenth week of pregnancy. She was accompanied by her husband, James.

When I called out Linda's name in our Dallas surgery center waiting room, a heavily tattooed couple in black biker leathers rose and walked to meet me, helmets in hand. Their necks and arms were covered in black vines sprouting skulls. When I caught my breath and offered my standard spiel on our protocol requiring me to meet first with the patient alone, they interlaced their free hands. "We're in this together. I want him with me," she pleaded.

James was nodding his head and looking from her to me. His eyes said *please*.

I assured them that I would include James as soon as possible, and they hugged goodbye at our security door. When Linda and I sat down in the counseling room and I explained our intent—to guard against coercion and ensure confidentiality—Linda's reply was immediate: "We've been married almost twenty years, and we've never had a secret from each other. He's the best father in the world. This is even harder on him than it is on me. We both know it's the right thing to do, but he's heartbroken. Plus, he's worried for me. We've never done this before."

I got the message and stepped out to invite James to join us.

"Oh, thank you!" he said as I shook his hand and introduced myself. "I wish I could go through this for her." They sat together on the small sofa in the counseling room and embraced. James then turned his attention to me and, with one hand on Linda's swollen belly, continued. "We'd have this baby if there was any way. Linda's so beautiful, but I swear she's even more beautiful when she's pregnant. Coming here is the hardest thing we've ever done . . . and we've had some hard times. I was out of work for a while, and we've worried about feeding our children. That's the worst. But I'm foreman of the construction crew now, and we bought our first home last year."

Linda picked up the story seamlessly. "The boys share one bedroom, and the girls share the other. They even have a bathroom. They've never had it so good. Neither have we—and we can't ruin it with another baby now. We're just making ends meet. Another child would take us all under. I wish I could have this one, but there's no way." James was rubbing Linda's belly the whole time, and their shared pain in letting this pregnancy go was plain to see.

Linda was eighteen weeks pregnant, instead of the more common eight to ten weeks, because they'd celebrated two of their children's birthdays since she realized she was pregnant, and marking their birthdays with parties had consumed their time and money. Now that the birthdays were behind them, they could attend to the abortion. They had no experience with abortion, no awareness that the process would now cost more, require two days, and carry greater medical risks for Linda. Although abortion at eighteen weeks remains safer than childbirth, the risks do increase with each week of pregnancy. But from their point of view, an abortion was an abortion, and it would be hard for them at any time.

They concluded our meeting with the comment that all James had to do was look at Linda to get her pregnant. He joked that they needed to store their toothbrushes in separate cups on the bathroom counter lest his toothbrush magically impregnate her again. They were sad and tender and funny, a delight to meet. I wished them well, and we discussed the possibility of permanent sterilization for one of them—medically easier for James and something he wanted to do since he couldn't have the abortion for Linda.

The following day, when we'd safely and successfully ended Linda's pregnancy, I found James in our parking lot. I told him the abortion was over and everything had gone well. He jumped up from the curb where he'd been sitting and threw his arms around me as he cried in relief.

I truly do not know what I expected when I took Curtis up on his offer to train abortion counselors—except that the task would be quick and easy. I never dreamed I would be counseling heavily tattooed parents of five. My world is expanded. I'm so glad I was wrong.

. . . .

I began with the arrogance of youth and an added dose of Glenna-the-know-it-all who would find her place in *The World Book Encyclopedia*. The work humbled me from day one, but the magic is that patients continue to surprise me. They not only challenge my professional skills; they force me to look within, revealing my prejudices and exposing my blind spots. I won't make the encyclopedia pages, but with many of our patients, I realize my alternate childhood ambition: to travel the world on the Good Ship *HOPE*.

Abortion counseling affords me an ongoing education. I engage in a meaningful way with people I might never meet in daily life, whose lives and cultures are so different from my own—and all as I work to make the world a safer place for women and their families. Learning from them enlarges my worldview.

We once saw a woman and her partner who lived in a garbage dump in Oklahoma. She had seen two other doctors who refused to provide care. Both doctors told her she was "too fat," but I suspect that equal, unspoken barriers were the fact that she and her partner are developmentally disabled—and had no money for care. Our clinics have a reputation among other providers for seeing so-called lost causes, which is probably why she'd been referred to us.

Her partner had borrowed an old, battered car and driven her to Dallas. Her obesity did make an accurate sonogram or pelvic exam impossible, but Curtis was moved by the couple's devotion to each other and their determination to solve their problem. So, he decided to trust her menstrual history and give this couple his best effort, reasoning that he could quit if the effort proved too risky. Fortunately, her internal anatomy allowed him to locate the pregnancy and easily terminate it.

I met the patient in the recovery room, where she was munching on Oreos and declaring them the best thing she'd ever eaten. When I told her that the doctor wanted her to know how well the procedure had gone, and that she could safely return to Oklahoma, she started to sob.

"You all are the first people who've treated me like I'm people," she said. "Tell that doctor I love him. He just saved our life."

CHAPTER TEN

Blessings: Faith, Acceptance, and Terminal Uncertainty

"I'm so grateful for having a choice. Thank you to everyone
who helped me here in this office! Blessing to all the women
who need this & to the people who take care of us!"
—*Patient journal entry*

Glenna

Our first blessing ceremony was unplanned—a surprising request from a patient. It was 1978 or '79, after Curtis and I had returned to work full-time in Dallas. I was counseling a patient named Janet, who was confident about her decision to end the pregnancy. Then she mentioned, as if it were an afterthought, that she wondered what the people at her church back home in Malakoff would think if they knew. I knew a bit about her small town near Curtis's homeplace in Athens—among "God's people," known to outsiders as the Texas Bible Belt—so I took note.

"How important is their opinion?" I asked.

"Oh, they'll never know, so I guess it doesn't matter."

But she'd brought it up, so there was something. "Have you talked with God about this?" I was betting on a deity. After all, she'd said church.

"Hmm . . . no," Janet replied.

"Do you usually talk things over with your god?" I asked.

"Sometimes, if I'm confused. But I'm not confused about this."

"Does God know you're here today?"

"He must," she said. "He sees everything."

"Then what do you believe He's thinking?"

"That I'm doing what's best for everyone."

That fit with what she'd told me. I suspected there was more to it—there always is—but she'd reaffirmed her decision. Instead of probing, I offered information I'd never shared with a patient before. "Your doctor today was a minister before he went to medical school. Many religious people support abortion, but I trust your judgment about whom to tell . . . and not tell."

She chuckled. "Yeah. Thanks." And we talked of other things.

Her eight-week abortion went smoothly, painlessly. Curtis joined me at the head of the table to let her know that all was well and say, "Goodbye. Call us if you need."

Then, as he left the room, Janet whispered, "Would he baptize my baby?"

Definitely something more, I thought, but I just said, "Let me ask him."

Daniece walked in to help Janet dress, and I slipped out to find Curtis in the lab, examining Janet's pregnancy with the magnifying glass. Translucent, shrimplike, and the size of the white tip of my little fingernail, it floated in a Pyrex dish backlit by the X-ray view box on the countertop. I touched his shoulder. "She wants you to baptize her baby."

"What?" His expression was quizzical, confused.

"Baptize the pregnancy."

"Is that kosher?"

I laughed. "The Baptist preacher asks the atheist if a blessing is kosher? Of course it is!"

"I'm not sure." He frowned. Curtis takes religion seriously.

"This isn't a joke, Curtis. She's asking you to bless her pregnancy. You're doing it for her," I insisted.

"But she'll never know."

"We will know. Please."

Curtis ran fresh water from the lab faucet—not the flowing stream of his youthful faith, but we were making do—and made the sign of the cross. "I bless you in the name of the Father, the Son, and the Holy Spirit," he said as he sprinkled tap water into the dish.

I returned to Janet, who was dressed and ready to go to the recovery room. "He baptized your pregnancy."

"Thank him," she replied, and something indefinable changed in her eyes as she repeated it. "Please, thank him for me."

I nodded. "You were wise to ask."

"Hmm. I don't know why. It just popped into my head after he said, 'Goodbye.'"

Later that day I did thank Curtis, telling him of Janet's visible relief.

As always, Curtis would ruminate on the experience and ponder the possibilities, and our routine patient care soon became more consciously ceremonial—not religious, but ceremonial. I started to recognize the routines we already observed as ritual elements in our "ceremony" of abortion. Every step in our process with each patient began taking on a deeper meaning for me.

There is a natural ritual to our first telephone contact with a patient—a literal one, in the list of facts to gather and instructions to give, but another one first: we listen. We introduce ourselves by name, use the patient's name, and ask about her concerns before we pelt her or her family or friend with questions. Curtis still remembers the first time he watched me on the phone, shocked as I gestured with my hands, my face animated as if in conversation with a real person in front of me. I'd grown up with a phone, while he had not; as a child, I had thought the operator was one of my invisible friends. And when talking with an invisible friend, tone of voice is key—we need to start by matching that of the caller, then shift to a warmer tone to develop a budding trust with the stranger at the other end of line.

Then at the reception desk, the patient and any companions need to meet a friendly face, not a bright, cheerful smile—that is probably not the patient's mood—but a warm one. When the counselor calls the patient from the waiting room, the same holds true: the counselor must first see the patient and observe her facial expression, posture, clothing, and grooming. Our counselors get their best initial sense of the patient while remaining open to what we hope will unveil in counseling.

With each step in the process, from counseling to the necessary lab work to the surgery area, the staff interact with warmth and respect for each other and for the patient as they pass her on. After the procedure, the nurse or medical assistant escorts the patient to recovery and makes an introduction as well as delivering the patient chart. The staff wish the patient well, say goodbye, and stop back to check on the patient if she is still there when they have occasion to return. There is a natural ritual to the steps in our process of delivering care, and valuing the rituals gives them greater meaning—consciously for staff and subliminally for patients.

. . . .

Although Curtis and I come from such different cultural and religious backgrounds, our humanitarian values, wide-ranging curiosities, and shared love for the natural world are our common ground. They have provided an instinctual bond that spills over from our personal to our professional lives and informs the rituals and blessings we continually create in both realms.

Having grown up without religious teaching, the importance of religion to many of our patients has been a revelation to me and opened a window into my own life. Throughout my secular childhood, I developed a fascination with anthropology and sociology, and by high school I was reading in both fields, searching for my intellectual home. I read for pleasure and on a journey to find answers to my lingering questions: *Where does the sun come from when it grows out of the hilltop at dawn, and where does it go at night? Who is the God my friends talk about? And where did my bird, Timmy, go when he died in Daddy's hands?*

Like most children, I wondered about nearly everything. When I asked Mother my endless questions, she took my curiosity seriously. When I was five or six, she showed me pictures from my *World Book* and gave one of her lectures on the solar system, so I knew the sun was looking at the other side of the earth at night, and I wanted to see those exotic places too. But she said God and Timmy's fate were matters of belief, and I should study anthropology to find those answers. She showed me her copy of *The Hero with a Thousand Faces*, by Joseph Campbell—one of her personal heroes—and took me to one of her sacred spaces, the Modesto Public Library, to find anthropology books. She helped me read the hard parts of the most important books and then explained stuff that got too confusing. Her explanations were the best part and no doubt fed my abiding interest in what other people believe and celebrate.

That curiosity has inspired my respect for our patients' beliefs, not because I share their beliefs but because I suspect their faith provides answers to the mysteries I have never been able to solve. I am someone who lives in what a physician friend once diagnosed as "terminal uncertainty." His joke was on the mark. I am a wonder-wanderer in my mind, in books, and in the world.

I have approached our patients' beliefs with genuine curiosity, explaining that I'm not of their faith but want to understand where abortion fits in their tradition. In New Mexico, we typically have a mix of Hispanic, Anglo, and Native American patients awaiting care. In Dallas, we have seen a wider range of Anglo American, African American, and varied Latinx patients, joined by new immigrant and refugee populations over the years—women from Africa and Asia, as well as Latin America.

For some of our patients, their religious and cultural traditions provide comfort and community. For others, like Nadia, religion and culture are also a source of shame and trauma.

Nadia was thirty-eight years old when I met her in Dallas. She had emigrated from Sudan at least twenty years earlier. She reported a college education in the United States and had filled out the paperwork with ease but was shy about speaking in English, apologizing that hers wasn't adequate. She worked as a statistical analyst at a tech company, so she was clearly intelligent and fluent in computer languages. In counseling, she struggled in apparent shame, her head bowed and her words choked out slowly, to tell me two important things.

First, she wanted to be tied down and blindfolded for the abortion. She desperately wanted to end the pregnancy but was afraid she would be unable to bear the pain. To explain that we never use physical restraints—as an act of respect for our patients and because the abortion is typically not painful—I used my stock comparison: "It's more like a pelvic exam that lasts a few minutes longer than usual."

Nadia shook her head. She'd never had a pelvic exam.

Wanting to reassure her that the abortion would not be as painful as she imagined, and stretching for a comparison, I asked if sexual intercourse was usually painful. She again bowed her head and found the words to tell me the second important thing: this pregnancy was the result of rape, and it had been very painful.

This time I had no words. When I offered my hand, she clutched it.

We completed the paperwork, and I escorted Nadia to the procedure room, where she changed into the medical gown. I explained that I would arrange her on the exam table and offered to do her first pelvic exam so she would know what to expect. She nodded, and I stepped to the end of the exam table to place her legs in the knee rests. That's when I saw the genital mutilation.

Nadia's clitoris was gone. What had once been the outer and inner lips of her vagina were a ragged mass of scar tissue. I had seen clitorectomies years earlier, when Dallas had experienced an influx of Ethiopian refugees in the 1980s, but even so, this level of damage was shocking to my eyes. I donned gloves, spoke in gentle tones, and proceeded slowly, describing each touch. Her rigid body slowly relaxed, and when I had the speculum in place, I asked if she wanted me to leave it inside so the doctor would not need to repeat the process.

"Please," she replied.

When Dr. Alan, who had waited patiently outside the door, walked in, Nadia panicked at the sight of him—a man. I stood beside as she again begged me to hold her down and blindfold her. Improvising, I pulled a tissue from the bedside box and draped it over her eyes, leaning my body over her in an embrace as she moaned her fear.

I watched as Dr. Alan—a West Texas cowboy in dress and speech, a kind and skilled ER doctor by training—registered the shock I had felt upon seeing the damage to her genital area. We nodded to each other. He completed her abortion in minutes and without pain. When he stood to say, "All done," Nadia pulled me even closer.

"I love you," she whispered as I wiped her tears with that tissue.

Most of our patients have not endured the horrors of Nadia's coming-of-age ritual, but I certainly know that more women have been raped or sexually violated in other ways than any public record will ever show. I can only hope that the way we performed Nadia's abortion offered a measure of healing for the trauma she lived through—both her ritual female circumcision and the violation of her recent rape.

Such experiences remind me that our histories are always with us, for better and for worse. Some bring peace and enlightenment, while others haunt the lives of our patients and our staff who spend time with them and their stories.

· · · ·

Part of the power of abortion counseling is the opportunity it affords patients, the chance to reexamine accepted beliefs and reveal what might otherwise remain secret. I suspected this from the start, but our patient journals confirmed my suspicion.

The journals are simple spiral notebooks from the back-to-school aisle at the supermarket. Since 2010, we have kept a journal beside each chair in our recovery rooms in both Texas and New Mexico. Typed on their cardboard or plastic covers is an invitation, "Please feel free to write whatever you would like in this journal—for yourself or for others." I have learned so much from what our patients write on those blank pages. As they recover or await their next procedure, they reflect. When patients speak for themselves, they express every one of this book's themes in hundreds of different ways and words. I love the handwriting, the errors in spelling and grammar, the emojis they draw, but most of all I love the immediacy of their feelings, the rawness captured on those pages.

The obvious belief our patients reexamine is their opinion on abortion—the deed, the sort of person who would have one, and the people who provide them. One patient wrote, "I used to judge/hate people who have had or are for abortions but now I see that in some situations an abortion may be the best choice for the unborn baby & the people in our lives so now I promise not to judge any one for their choice. I don't know their feelings or situation but now I feel their hurt. I thank ALL the staff for kindness & comfort they gave me through the hardest choice I ever had in my life."[39]

She signs this entry "Heartbroken." This is not a young teen writing; she is a twenty-nine-year-old mother of four, and this abortion has taught her what Christians call the Golden Rule: *Do unto others as you would have them do unto you.* And like all of us, she had to learn it the hard way—through humility.

Another patient spoke for so many others when she wrote, "As I sit here with so many emotions, I read this book with [entries by] women who come from all walks of life having to make the same decision I've just made. A sense of relief has set into my heart for I know I'll never feel alone."[40] Feeling "not alone" is vital to this woman because the story she then tells is a story of navigating life alone, the story of so many of the women we see: "I'm a single mother already. I couldn't do this alone. At least not right now."

She explains that the man who impregnated her has left her. "We were so happy about our baby, planning our future together . . . I want my children to have a better life than I [had. To be] emotionally, spiritually, loved, wanted, all the things I never had. I want to let whoever is reading this know we all have been there, but it's our choice. I feel guilty but I know I didn't want to bring my baby into a broken life. I'm broken. . . . It wouldn't have been fair. I will never forget today. But I will move on and make things better. I'm sorry my baby. Please forgive me." Many of our patients sign their journal entries "Mommy." This woman simply leaves her initials.

We have years of journals from both Dallas and Albuquerque, and each entry speaks a near-universal truth. In the margins, patients write to each other as if in meditative conversation. One entry begins with a drawing of a heart with a lightning bolt splitting it. Below the symbol, the patient states, "I pray God will forgive me for doing this, but I feel he will understand that as a mother I did what was best for my child." Below this another hand has written, "God will forgive you and bless you forever!" In the margin a third has added, "God will always love you."

In these difficult moments, our patients see beyond themselves, reaching out to each other—treating others as they want to be treated themselves—practicing the Golden Rule.

As I learned in my first week on the job, humility is not only a virtue; it is a necessity in caring for others. And like the Golden Rule, we learn it backward—coming to humility by recognizing our own errors, to the Golden Rule by accepting our own needs.

For providers as well as patients, soul searching is not required, but it is on offer.

· · · ·

In contrast to Curtis's early life, the real sanctuary in my childhood was never a church or even a library. It was nature. As a young girl, I absorbed a wordless sense of the sacred and a love of family rituals that, later in life, opened me up to our patients' spiritual needs.

Every spring we made a family pilgrimage to Yosemite to see the dogwood trees in bloom and have a picnic in the woods as our birthday gift to my mother. We went camping every summer, and we took weekend trips throughout the year to walk the sand dunes at Big Sur or stand in silent awe among the giant sequoias near Three Rivers. When Mother died, she left a list of all these places and more, so we could spread her ashes in the perfect spots for her "eternal rest." Daddy did not leave instructions for after his death, but Eddy and I knew where to spread his—mostly close to Mother's.

Our first ritual spreading of Mother's ashes was in our backyard. On my parents' last trip to New Mexico together, they spent hours sitting on our back patio, watching the birds that nest in our trees and bathe in our small pond. They shared a pair of binoculars, and Mother had *Peterson's Field Guide to the Birds of North America* on her lap. Roger Tory Peterson was another one of her heroes, and I remembered the book from childhood—it went everywhere with us in her overstuffed handbag. That afternoon, Mother looked up when I joined them and said, "If I had another life to live, I think I'd be an ornithologist."

We had no idea that her own death was approaching, but something guided me to say, "Yes, you would have loved that." And then I—who had always cringed when she spoke of being cremated—said, "We'll spread some of your ashes by the pond, so I know you're here watching the birds."

"I'd like that," she said.

And so we did.

We built an altar to Mary, beloved mother and grandmother, on the big flat rock at the end of the pond. A studio portrait from when she was young and gorgeous, and my snapshot of her in death—a death mask—were lit by candles in two of her silver candlesticks. We spread her ashes and blew out the candles, and her six-year-old granddaughter, Casey, determined to be a big girl, was so proud when she made it through the ceremony without tears. As it grew dark, we gathered up the sacred articles from Mary's altar. Casey wanted to help and, in the process, skinned her knee on the rock—just a minor abrasion, but she howled, and all her unshed tears followed. Yes, one of the powers of ritual is to relieve our grief.

When I had my cancer surgery, I made a different sort of altar on the bedside shelf in my hospital room: photos of my mother and dreaded grandmother, who had both survived breast cancer when it was considered fatal; my treasured Elmer the elephant from infancy, my equivalent of the well-worn Velveteen Rabbit and missing one button eye; flowers from special friends; the Magic Slate our friend Emerson brought so I could communicate in writing long before I could talk again. The nurses and aides all stared at my shelf of curiosities. As they got to know me and finally asked about that shelf, I used that Magic Slate to tell the story of my Altar to Survival.

If they thought I was nuts, they had the grace not to say so.

To this day, I build altars in our home for those I love whenever they are in need. Years later, when a Buddhist couple arrived in the clinic, asking to set up an altar with flowers and fruit in the procedure room, I immediately understood their need. I cleansed the instrument tray and its stand, draped it, and left them to create their altar.

Hopefully, we all have our rituals and are grateful for our many blessings.

Curtis

Christian faith, the King James Bible, and our one-room church in the woods—these were at the center of my life as a child. For three weeks out of the month, our old wooden-plank church was unoccupied. Maybe a few people visited family members buried in its cemetery, but not often. The old building was tucked away on a plot of land my grandfather had donated to the church, half a mile from the nearest farmhouse—a sacred, silent space. But on the third Sunday of every month and, as in Old Testament tradition, the Saturday beforehand, that old building became the center of our world. It was transformed into a sanctuary.

People came by car, by foot, or—in my grandmother's time—by wagon. Many stayed overnight, bunking with relatives or friends. By Friday night, the preachers would arrive—one or two of the four itinerant preachers who served eight churches scattered over several counties—and we'd welcome them like royalty. The double doors of the church swung open Saturday morning and didn't shutter again until Sunday night. The otherwise silent building rang with voices raised in prayer, testimony, and song.

In so many ways I am light-years away from that place and the religion I was raised in, but I still have fond memories of sitting next to my grandmother on the wooden pew, nestled against her full bosom as her fan whipped the warm air against my face. Even as a child, I had questions the ministers couldn't answer, but I never questioned my community. This was home. I knew that if my family ever needed help bringing in the harvest or caring for the livestock, our church family would be there, just as we were there for them. Such was our code: if a brother or sister asks for help, you help.

After two and a half days of food, gossip, services, and song, it would be time to say goodbye. The preacher would lead us in a hymn. We had no musical instruments, and anyway, our hymnal didn't have musical notes—only the words, and we knew them all by heart:

> *My Christian Friends in bonds of love,*
> *Whose hearts in sweetest union join,*
> *Your friendship's like a drawing band,*
> *Yet we must take the parting hand.*

As they sang, people moved about the sanctuary, embracing, kissing each other on the cheek, even on the lips. Men and women mixed together, smiling and crying. The song speaks of the sorrow of parting and the bonds of love that connect us. The power of this stays with me even now:

> *Your company's sweet,*
> *Your union dear,*
> *Your words delightful to my ear,*
> *Yet when I see that we must part,*
> *You draw like cords around my heart.*

I loved these people, and I knew they cared for me, but as my religious doubts grew, I was torn. When they would say, "Brother, you're going to be a great preacher someday," I continued to reply, "If God wills." But as I grew older, the meaning of that stock reply changed. Perhaps God had a different plan for me.

In the end, I left my faith, but I'd like to think that the best of my faith stayed with me. Undoubtedly, I took with me its code of service. And I still cherish the feelings of brotherly love and belonging that came with our ritual greetings and farewells. Perhaps unconsciously, I have spent much of my adult life seeking that feeling again. Alone and unsupported, I could not have endured in this work for over fifty years. Everyone needs and deserves to feel worthy in themselves—and to be a part of something greater than themselves.

Before *Roe*, I was isolated by necessity. So were many of the women who came to me for help, in secret, often without support even from partners, let alone communities. Among my first generation of patients, those who came to me through the Clergy Consultation Service had better outcomes, but not because they received religious counsel. In fact, the clergy were not permitted to impose their own views on abortion or religion on the women who came to them. As devoted to their own faiths as many of the clergy were, their purpose was simply to help women—regardless of their own faith—get to and from medically trained abortion providers safely. That they did so without judgment was their greatest service. They delivered these women into a sense of community.[41]

All women served by the CCS gained reassurance that the doctor to whom they were referred could be trusted, but also that they themselves were still good people, and—by the symbolic power of referral through a spiritual leader—that their decision was acceptable in God's eyes, regardless of what they may have heard from the pulpit of their own church. They need not feel estranged from their god and a larger community of love and faith.

As much as I respected the clergy of the CCS and valued their protection and support, we worked at a distance, so for me, they could provide only a limited sense of community. But as I discovered, the sense of acceptance and community that all humans need does not have to come from religion. Ultimately, I found the love and the support I needed in Glenna, and I found community in the wonderful staff we have created and re-created throughout our career together.

. . . .

Glenna and I already understood how important the total clinic environment was to the patients' experience, even before we introduced guided meditation for pain management into our practice in the late 1970s. During surgeries, we routinely turned down the lights, turned on soothing music, and spoke in soft tones. We kept quiet, calm, and attentive, creating a serene atmosphere so the patient could relax. But we wanted something more.

We wanted patients to leave feeling better about themselves, empowered by their ability to make an important decision and by the respect with which we treated them. We wanted our clinic to provide a community of safety and acceptance—to be a secular sanctuary.

My childhood immersion in the church encourages me to think of each element of our work in terms of ceremony and ritual. Framing our entire abortion service as ceremonial helps ground us in staying mindful and present for whatever comes. Ceremony does not dictate experience; it makes space for it.

In my mind, the ceremony is the whole, and the rituals are its components. Although the whole process appears routine, prosaic, to me it has always felt poetic, like the lines in our church hymnal. And as with poetry, our patients don't need to understand it to be moved.

So it is at the clinic too. Patients may not realize that the walls in the waiting room are painted in subtle shades of blue and purple, colors known to inspire calm and even lower blood pressure. They may not notice the art on the walls, or the way the chairs and couches are arranged in intimate groupings rather than clinical rows, but we hope the environment makes them feel less anxious all the same.

For me, the most meaningful rituals are those of greeting and farewell. I meet the patient one-on-one while she is still in her street clothes, not undressed and reclining on the exam table. We sit facing each other on chairs of the same height, as a matter of respect. I take care to look her in the eye as we talk. Our meeting may be brief, but in this way, I let her know: *I see you as a person first and a patient second. I am listening and attentive to your needs.* Any medical student who trains with me, and any doctor who works for me, practices this ritual.

After the procedure, I go to the head of the table and say my farewell. The patient may be groggy from the medications, but I touch her shoulder gently to make contact. If she responds, I offer her my hand. "We are all finished here. Everything went well," I say. "How did it go for you?"

Anyone watching would not know that this leave-taking is part of our abortion ceremony. Patients aren't told about our philosophy. It is meaningless to say, *I am going to be kind to you.* Just do it. Do it for everyone, no exceptions.

Finally, I remind her that she can contact us with any concerns. "Call any time," I say. It is a farewell, but with a promise of continued connection if she wants or needs it. In this way, I extend the "parting hand" of that heartfelt hymn.

. . . .

Both Glenna and I believe that our ceremonial approach to abortion allowed Janet to feel safe asking for a baptism—I had just offered her my parting hand. Yet despite my philosophy of patient-centered care and my wish to accommodate patients' special needs, I was caught unprepared.

Glenna was free to hear Janet's request as a basic human need for a ritual of closure, a recognition of her experience that expressed her regard for her pregnancy. But my own religious background and beliefs about what baptism means and how it is traditionally performed were in the way. When Glenna translated "baptism" as "blessing" and reminded me that it would be for the patient, I understood. I blessed that aborted pregnancy with the words of baptism as I knew them. And then, as Glenna surmised, I pondered the possibilities.

To our knowledge, no other abortion provider has offered blessings at their clinics. Years later, George Tiller would employ a minister to address patients' religious needs, but in the late 1970s, we were outliers. We wondered: How could—or should—we offer this ritual?

We did not want to impose a spiritual component on anyone who would not choose it. We knew the patient who had asked for that first blessing felt more at peace afterward. Would it have been even more powerful if we had been in the room with her? Would other patients want a blessing if they knew it was available to them?

We talked with the staff, and most were intrigued by the idea. As a group, we decided that if a patient seemed to be struggling spiritually or emotionally, the counselor could offer a blessing. We weren't sure anyone would even make such a request.

To our surprise, many did.

Blessings, like guided meditations, are patient-led. Some patients, like Janet, want to bless the fetus, to say goodbye with love. Some pray for the fetus to return later, when they are better able to care for it. Others want to receive the blessing, to make peace with themselves or their higher power. We don't presume to know what patients want. We simply talk with each patient who wants a blessing before surgery to learn her wishes.

Most blessings have elements in common. Generally, we place the pregnancy in a small silver bowl and wrap it in blue medical paper from the lab. The counselor brings the bowl into the room while the lights are still low. She hands the bowl to me, and I offer it to the patient. I invite her to place one hand below the bowl and one above. I place my hands over hers. We bow our heads, and the words follow.

Often our patients provide the words in the form of a poem, a letter, even a song for the occasion. Some recite favorite prayers. Others prefer silence. Some want their partners or other family to be present. I usually request the presence of the counselor and nurse, but sometimes the patient or family members prefer that we are not involved.

They may bring tokens of their faith or perform ceremonies from their own traditions.

I have facilitated many blessings, but one stands out to me above the others. One of our counselors, an artist, had prepared a third-trimester fetus with great aesthetic care—swaddling it in a doll-size blanket and nesting the bundle in a small wicker basket we use for this purpose. The patient and her family had traveled a great distance to end this longed-for pregnancy. A fetal defect, incompatible with life, had been detected late in pregnancy, and the entire family was heartbroken. What I remember is how our patient cradled her fetus in its basket, how she whispered against its ear, kissed its cheeks. She passed the basket to her partner, who pressed it to his chest and spoke softly. He passed the bundle first to his mother and then to hers. Each parent and grandparent had a chance to stroke a cheek or kiss miniature fingers.

It was the ritual of the parting hand.

That old feeling of community from my childhood church rose up in me as we embraced one another, saying farewell. Medically speaking, this family was holding a fetus. A baby has to be born alive and breathe on its own. But emotionally, to this family, they were saying goodbye to their baby and demonstrating the bonds of love, not only for their aborted pregnancy but for each other. They would not just survive this loss; they would be stronger for it.

Many patients send us cards or letters to thank us and to share what was most meaningful to them about their time with us. If they had a blessing ritual, that experience usually tops their list.[42] The other thing patients consistently note is that they've never before been to a medical facility where everyone is noticeably kind to them.

I'm sorry to hear of those other experiences but pleased as well. I want patients to have good memories, just as I want to have good memories of our patients and their experiences. This gives me great comfort and satisfaction. It's what I want for myself, for our staff, and for the women we serve. And if that is what we want, then we must begin each patient interaction with this end in mind.

. . . .

Words haven't always come easily to me. As a teen, when my grandmother thought I might one day be a preacher, I struggled to pin down what often felt like a whirlwind of questions and ideas. Fortunately, our old church didn't believe in scripted testimony. It was acceptable to wait until the spirit moved you to speak. I learned to wait.

But sometimes there are no words. In times of great joy or sorrow, what we *do* matters far more than what we *say*. Perhaps this explains why ceremony and ritual remain important to me, and to Glenna too. Even now, so many years after I left the church, I still believe that through mindful action, it is possible to convey true depth of feeling.

I look back with fondness to some of the rituals from my youth, and perhaps the most meaningful was the one for which our Primitive Baptist Church received its nickname "foot-washing Baptists." The ritual is based on the biblical story of Jesus bending to wash the feet of his disciples at the Last Supper. Foot washing was a job for servants. By bowing before his followers to wash their feet, Jesus embodied humility and leadership through service.

Likewise, before our church services ended and we prepared to part, male members of the congregation would bow before other men; women would bow before other women. In turns, we would wash each other's feet. Without words—or beyond them—we told one another that we are each other's caretakers and that each of us is deserving of care. One need not believe in a god to appreciate the symbolic power of such a ritual.

I loved and admired the people of my childhood community, but I also struggled to fully understand them. They were hardworking folks who would do anything to help a neighbor. But these same people might also shun an unmarried pregnant woman or insist that a person of color drink from a separate water fountain. We are told to be good people who do good work, but what does that really mean? One person's good might be another's sin.

I am well aware that what I consider good work is believed to be sinful by others. They can think what they like of me. But I will not accept their demeaning caricatures of women who seek abortions. With broad strokes, they paint two-dimensional pictures of women as selfish, promiscuous, anti-child, anti-man "feminazis," or as innocent victims duped into terminating their pregnancies by predatory abortionists. This is insulting to women and families and abortion providers alike.

For the record, although our clinics have performed well over half a million abortions, I am not pro-abortion. Many abortion providers would say the same.

I am pro-woman.

I trust women to know their lives, needs, strengths, and limits. Choosing whether to continue or end a pregnancy is a private and—in my opinion—highly ethical decision-making process. Most women consider not just how a pregnancy would affect their lives but how their current life circumstances could affect the well-being of a child. In my experience, women choose to have abortions because they value the potential life they carry.

Glenna and I believe that the struggle toward justice and liberty for all—including women—is the right thing to do and that it is an eternal struggle. Neither of us believes in a deity, but we can speak to how healing it is to be truly present for one another in times of grief and growth and change. We are fortunate to have worked with extraordinary doctors, nurses, counselors, and office staff who hold similar values and who are present in the same way for each other. We are naturally biased in thinking that ours is a special group, but the truth is that abortion providers are among the most compassionate people we have ever met. We are grateful to be members of that community.

I may have fond memories of my childhood church, but I could not return to it now. I am not the same person I was as a boy sitting on that old wooden pew next to my grandmother. While I take with me a deep appreciation for ceremony and ritual from my past, I cannot accept the widespread prejudice and bigotry so evident among religious fundamentalists today.

Even as a medical student, I struggled to reconcile my unease with the church with my love for my people. I ultimately left the church before I left my community, and I found myself among the Unitarian Universalists—a church group known for accepting all, including the spiritual diaspora from traditional religions. Eventually, I would call myself a spiritual atheist, a secular humanist, but at the time I did not know where I fit between the seemingly conflicting worlds of science and faith—until I sat on a pew in the First Unitarian Church of Dallas, listening and feeling moved by the closing words of the Unitarian benediction.

We ask these things in the name of all helpers of humankind.

I did not know then where my life's path would lead. I could not have imagined that I would perform abortions or that one day I would marry Glenna. But if I could have imagined it, I would've hoped only that together we would devote our lives to doing exactly what we have done: providing abortions in the service of women's equal place in society and, with our staff, holding a place among the helpers of humankind.

Afterword

"There remains for us only the very narrow way, often extremely difficult to find, of living every day as if it were our last, and yet living in faith and responsibility as though there were to be a great future."
—*Dietrich Bonhoeffer*

Glenna

Although we have finished writing this book, our work remains unfinished. When the goal is social change, that is a given. Yet in the case of access to safe, legal abortion, much of what Curtis and I created has been undone by larger social and political movements in the United States today.

This book mirrors our life in its intentional focus on the needs of our patients and the reality of providing abortion care within our clinic walls, *not* the struggle for the right to legal abortion, nor the ever-escalating harassment and violence. That story has been recorded in the daily news. We have recounted such events only as they have touched us directly, recalling the feminist slogan of the 1970s: "The Personal Is Political."

We wanted to ground our collective understanding of abortion in reality, not slogans. We chose to tell personal stories—our own and our patients'—because in the political war against abortion that has raged since the 1980s, the deep and varied meaning of abortion in the lives of real people has been lost.

Obviously, we began writing long before June 24, 2022, when the Supreme Court ruled on *Dobbs v. Jackson Women's Health Organization*. That decision overturned the fifty-year-old *Roe v. Wade* ruling by declaring that the US Constitution does not protect a woman's legal right to abortion. Each state is now at liberty to determine whether abortion is legal within its borders. Yet again the ground shifted, reminding us that, with abortion, the political truly is personal.

Curtis and I were at the Dallas surgery center when the decision was released. Our phones started to ring—both the office lines and our personal cell phones—as our attorneys and allies called to share their outrage and offer condolence. Curtis and I walked the surgery center halls in a daze, embracing our loyal staff. Then we huddled with our beloved co-directors in the administrative office to silently read the text of the decision. It was a long, surreal moment for all of us. "This feels like a death," I confessed. "I knew it was coming, yet I'm not prepared."

· · · ·

The consequences for our patients and our staff were too painful to voice. Curtis and I were the only people in the building who had been alive before *Roe*. For everyone else, our patients as well as staff, abortion had *always* been safe and legal.

Texas was poised to void all rights to abortion within its borders, and in compliance with Texas law, we saw our last abortion patient at Southwestern Women's Surgery Center in Dallas on August 24, 2022. The state now seeks to prosecute residents who obtain an abortion outside state borders and anyone who aids them in doing so. The clinic in New Mexico remains open, and every day its staff hears the desperate stories of women from Texas and other states with increasingly restrictive abortion laws.

In the days and weeks immediately following the *Dobbs* decision, I was devastated. I asked myself, *Why did we bother?* Not only with the years of daily work, from which we are now retired, but with writing about it *now*.

Of course, I knew the answer, but at the time that did not assuage my despair. Abortion has been with us "since the dawn of time." It will not go away. Thus, we write to support all the people whose lives have been touched by abortion—either their own or that of someone they love. You are not alone! In fact, you are in good company.

We write to share our experience with those who are conflicted and confused about the abortion issue. Again, you are not alone, and you too are in good company.

Finally, we write to leave a firsthand record for those who will continue to work for women's equal place in American society. And I am eternally grateful to those who follow us in this quest. The story of abortion after *Dobbs* will be another story—one which you will live to tell.

Despite the truth of this answer, I was troubled by another deeply personal question: Knowing how my career seems to end, do I wish I had chosen a different path?

In my mind's eye I see my mother sitting on our back patio wondering if she should have been an ornithologist. I chose a career in legal abortion services because I needed meaningful work, but also because—after learning hard lessons in systemic racism during the effort to desegregate Dallas's public schools—I needed a "win." Clearly, I do not end my career with a win, but years of work with abortion patients have taught me a very different lesson: The importance of tolerating our losses.

I wish my sense of loss were purely personal, but it is so much larger, and I don't yet have the larger words. I set out to change the world. I chose to do it one woman, one family, at a time. It has been slow going, and I end my career in profound sadness.

But life, and our patients, have taught me the small words that have become my personal consolation: This is the path I chose, and I have given it my best. I have learned and grown, both professionally and personally.

I would do it all over again.

Curtis

One evening, a few months after the Supreme Court decision that reversed *Roe*, Glenna and I sat on our back patio at home, looking out on the garden, the small pond where her mother's ashes rest, and the landscape beyond. To the west, we watched the sun draw low over the Jemez Mountains. To the east, we saw the Sangre de Cristo Mountains were upholding the promise of their Spanish name, glowing red like the "blood of Christ." That particular evening, the sunset painted the mountains mauve, and in their beauty and their grandeur, we each felt small, insignificant.

We were despondent over the *Dobbs* decision, which had just reversed *Roe v. Wade. Back where we began in the 1960s,* I thought. Our Dallas surgery center was closed, our life's work undone. None of it had made a difference in the end.

Then, reading each other's minds as we often do, we looked at each other and saw a glimmer of hope.

No! We were not back in the 1960s or in the Middle Ages, as some have declared. Much headway has been made, and that progress remains: Abortion will continue to be legal in about half of US states. Groups reminiscent of the CCS, the Janes, and others that sprung up in the 1960s and early '70s will continue organizing to help women get the care they need. And today, abortifacient pills can be mailed, bringing safe abortion to the homes of many who need it.

But I have an even deeper hope: What if the Supreme Court has kicked the hornets' nest with this decision?

I have vivid memories of kicking those nests on my childhood walks in the East Texas woods, and then fleeing the swarm of angry hornets. I believe that is what has happened with the Supreme Court decision. Aroused and angry, groups of citizens are now determined that women's rights shall not be erased.

A new awareness seems to have dawned on many people, which is all Glenna and I have ever wanted: the acknowledgment that whatever our beliefs—or yours—each woman should be able to decide for herself. They shall not have others' beliefs forced upon them—upon their lives and their bodies. The decision to continue or end a pregnancy must rest with the pregnant woman.

Finally, I also experienced a revelation: This is what democracy is about. We want—and therefore must tolerate—different opinions and beliefs in order to have a pluralistic society that functions. That principle is so simple in words, yet so hard to maintain.

So I implore the young people of our country to continue the quest for a better and fairer society for all, to secure full freedom and participation in all aspects of life for all people. And after fifty years, look back to see if you have accomplished some of your dreams. Then, decide if you have been fortunate enough to have made a difference.

That evening on the back patio, Glenna and I looked into each other's eyes, and I confirmed what we both knew.

Yes. We have made a difference.

Acknowledgments

This book has four godmothers: Caroline Little, Patricia O'Connor, Nan Ray, and Deborah Suder. Without the unique contributions of each of these remarkable women, we would not, perhaps could not, have written it.

We are blessed with the publisher, Kris Pauls, and editor, Alli Shapiro, of our dreams.

We are further blessed with more loyal friends, family, staff, and colleagues than we can name. They read raggedy drafts, providing the criticism and encouragement that guided and sustained us, while tolerating our neglect.

We are grateful—beyond words—to each and all of you.

Notes

1. The NYC group doing this same work proudly used the name Clergy Consultation Service on Abortion as a rejection of the stigmatization of the word, but I knew the Dallas group by this more euphemistic name.

2. Carole E. Joffe, *Doctors of Conscience: The Struggle to Provide Abortion Before and After Roe v. Wade* (Boston: Beacon Press, 1993), 29. I am indebted to Joffe for the phrase "doctors of conscience" in the title of her book on abortion providers who performed prelegal abortions and went on to work in the field after abortion became legal in the United States. Her phrase is an apt description of a number of abortion providers—both prelegal and since.

3. I have intentionally used the stigmatized term "abortionist" to denote my pride in having performed abortions before they were legalized. The pejorative term implied that the abortion provider was not a real doctor. I was a licensed MD with a thriving family practice when I chose to care for the patients I describe in this chapter.

4. Kristin Walter, "Early Pregnancy Loss," *JAMA*, https://jamanetwork.com/journals/jama/fullarticle/2803834.

5. These states were Georgia, Maryland, Arkansas, Delaware, Kansas, and New Mexico.

6. Willard Cates Jr., David A. Grimes, Kenneth F. Schulz, "Abortion Surveillance at CDC: Creating Public Health Light Out of Political Heat," *American Journal of Preventive Medicine* 19, S1 (2000):

S12–17, https://www.sciencedirect.com/science/article/abs/pii
/S0749379700001689.

7. My recollection of this quote was slightly off, but Skinner did discuss his grandmother's social climbing in several autobiographical works, now unfortunately out of print.

8. W. Bradford Wilcox, "The Evolution of Divorce," *National Affairs*, June 2009, https://nationalaffairs.com/publications/detail/the -evolution-of-divorce. Casey E. Copen, Kimberly Daniels, Jonathan Vespa, William D. Mosher, "First Marriages in the United States: Data from the 2006–2010 National Survey of Family Growth," *National Health Stat Report* 49 (March 2012): 1–21.

9. The rate is falling to about one in four with more effective long-acting contraceptives—and now with lack of access to legal abortion. However, during the years I was counseling patients, the one-in-three statistic held true. Rachel K. Jones, Jenna Jerman, "Abortion Incidence and Service Availability in the United States, 2011," *Perspectives on Sexual and Reproductive Health* 46 (March 2014): 3–14, https://pubmed .ncbi.nlm.nih.gov/24494995/. Margot Sanger-Katz, Claire Cain Miller, and Quoctrung Bui, "Who Gets Abortions in America?," *The New York Times*, December 14, 2021, https://www.nytimes.com /interactive/2021/12/14/upshot/who-gets-abortions-in-america.html.

10. "A Religious Right to Abortion: Legal History and Analysis," *Columbia Law School Center for Gender & Sexuality Law, Law Rights, and Religion Project*, August 2022, https://scholarship.law.columbia.edu/cgi /viewcontent.cgi?article=1017&context=gender_sexuality_law.

11. We are indebted to a personal communication with the scholar Gillian Frank, PhD, on July 10, 2023, for an understanding of the shared values as well as regional differences in pastoral care provided by the CCS. Casting abortion as "the lesser sin" was not common across the country, but it is my memory of the particular guide that I read.

12. "Safety of Abortion in the United States," *Advancing New Standards in Reproductive Health*, December 2014, https://www.ansirh.org/sites /default/files/publications/files/safetybrief12-14.pdf

13. Roberta Springer Loewy, "Women in Medicine: Recognition and Responsibility," *AMA Journal of Ethics*, July 2008, https://journalofethics.ama-assn.org/article/women-medicine-recognition-and-responsibility/2008-07. "Figure 12. Percentage of U.S. Medical School Graduates by Sex, Academic Years 1980–1981 Through 2018–2019," *Association of American Medical Colleges Diversity in Medicine: Facts and Figures 2019*, https://www.aamc.org/data-reports/workforce/data/figure-12-percentage-us-medical-school-graduates-sex-academic-years-1980-1981-through-2018-2019.

14. Uta Landy, Philip D. Darney, and Jody Steinauer, eds., *Advancing Women's Health Through Medical Education: A Systems Approach to Family Planning and Abortion* (Cambridge: Cambridge University Press, 2021).

15. Maureen Paul, ed., *A Clinician's Guide to Medical and Surgical Abortion* (New York: Churchill Livingstone, 1999), 86–7. I also contributed to the Counseling chapter in that text. Maureen Paul, ed., *Management of Unintended and Abnormal Pregnancy: Comprehensive Abortion Care* (Chichester, UK; Hoboken, NJ: Wiley-Blackwell, 2009), 101–3.

16. Herbert J. Freudenberger, "Staff Burn-Out," *Journal of Social Issues* 30 (Winter 1974): 159–65. Christina Maslach, "Burned-Out," *Human Behavior* 5 (September 1976): 16–22.

17. The origin of the term "burnout" was a late-night observation of the behavior of drug addicts in the NYC Bowery with whom the exhausted Herbert Freudenburger was working. A dedicated, and by all accounts driven, psychiatrist, Freudenburger would finish a long day of work with his Upper East Side patients and then spend hours volunteering in the Bowery, where he observed spaced-out addicts hold their cigarettes, to which they were also addicted, between their tobacco-stained fingers, oblivious as the cigarettes burned out and burned them in the process. Freudenberg realized that the image captured the state of the drug addicts but also that of the psychiatrist who wished to help them. Of course, burnout has become a more mainstream topic in the decades since I first began thinking about it, particularly in medicine and teaching.

18. Glenna's speech here is paraphrased from our memories. Our VCR tapes of the television coverage were destroyed in a fire years later, but it wouldn't have mattered. The segment that eventually aired featured a voiceover from the reporter while footage of Glenna's impromptu speech played silently in the background.

19. William Cates Jr., Charles Boyd, Glenna Halvorson-Boyd, Susan Holck, Thomas F. Gilchrist, "Death from Amniotic Fluid Embolism and Disseminated Intravascular Coagulation after a Curettage Abortion," *American Journal of Obstetrics and Gynecology* 141, no. 3 (October 1981): 346–48. Due to our immediate transparency with the CDC and Dallas Coroner's Office, this was the first autopsy-proven fatal case of AFE from abortion in the United States and provided the medical profession with valuable insight.

20. Glenna had been appalled by the worldwide success of the song "Evil Woman" by ELO (Electric Light Orchestra), released in 1975 and topping worldwide popular music charts by 1976. We were in our mountaintop retreat years, which gave her time to pay attention to such things, and she took note that the title was reviewed as such a successful hook line. I had no interest in the music of the time and could not understand her reaction. I saw it as irrelevant to abortion, and in explicit content it was. Her life experiences as a woman attuned her to the broader implications—particularly the view of women as the keepers of the virtues bestowed by the Lord and as subject to banishment if they did not keep those virtues intact. From Glenna's point of view "Evil Woman" was *The Scarlet Letter* in 1970s pop rock form.

21. S. Schneider, *Mademoiselle*, April 1968.

22. Joanmarie Kalter, "TV News and Religion: Network Coverage of Abortion," *TV Guide*, November 9, 1985.

23. "FBI Analysis of Terrorist Incidents in the United States, 1983," *U.S. Department of Justice Office of Justice Programs*, https://www.ojp.gov/ncjrs/virtual-library/abstracts /fbi-analysis-terrorist-incidents-united-states-1983.

24. For more on this, I highly recommend the CNN interview with Frank Schaeffer, a filmmaker whose father, Francis Schaeffer, was

instrumental in bringing Jerry Falwell to the anti-abortion movement. Frank later left the anti-abortion right and speaks candidly about his regret around furthering his father's work. "Why This Former Anti-abortion Activist Regrets the Movement He Helped Build," video, 19:46, CNN, May 4, 2022, YouTube, https://www.youtube.com /watch?v=25JyC5Whhvc.

25. Mirielle Jacobson and Heather Royer, "Aftershocks: The Impact of Clinic Violence on Abortion Services," *National Bureau of Economic Research*, December 2010, https://www.nber.org/papers/w16603.

26. The Ethical Principles of Professional-Patient Relationships are Veracity, at number one, followed by Fidelity, Privacy, and Confidentiality. A breach of any of these is grounds for disciplinary action. Ruth F. Craven and Constance J. Hirnle, eds., *Fundamentals of Nursing: Human Health and Function* (Philadelphia: Lippincott, Williams & Wilkins, 2003), 93.

27. Simon McCormack, "After the Fire: An Abortion Clinic Overcomes Arson with Resolve," *Weekly Alibi News*, January 31, 2008, https://alibi .com/news/after-the-fire/.

28. We are indebted to Joan for so many things, including access to her notes from the sentencing.

29. "Provider Security," *National Abortion Federation*, https://prochoice .org/our-work/provider-security/.

30. "Provider Security," *National Abortion Federation*.

31. Personal telephone communications with Jeanne Tiller on August 9, 2023, and August 13, 2023.

32. For more information and, of course, the opportunity to contribute to this fund, which is administered through the Wichita Community Foundation, see www.wichitacf.org. Most of the causes this dedicated fund supports are based in Kansas and include sex education for boys as well as girls.

33. Personal communication with Dr. Carter on July 11, 2023.

34. In fact, there were three abortion-related deaths in 2017 and between seven hundred and nine hundred deaths with childbirth. Correcting for the denominators, the ratio is essentially six hundred

maternal deaths with childbirth to one with abortion. Jeff Diamant and Besheer Mohamed, "What the Data Says about Abortion in the U.S.," *Pew Research Center*, January 11, 2023, https://www.pewresearch .org/short-reads/2023/01/11/what-the-data-says-about-abortion-in -the-u-s-2/. Donna L. Hoyert, "Maternal Mortality Rates in the United States, 2021," *Centers for Disease Control and Prevention National Center for Health Statistics*, https://www.cdc.gov/nchs/data/hestat/maternal -mortality/2021/maternal-mortality-rates-2021.htm#Table.

35. For more information on the demographics of abortion patients, see the Guttmacher Institute at www.guttmacher.org/united-states/abortion.

36. George Devereux, *A Study of Abortion in Primitive Societies: A Typological, Distributional, and Dynamic Analysis of the Prevention of Birth in 400 Pre-industrial Societies* (New York: The Julian Press, 1955).

37. This practice was discontinued in abortion care in the United States as medical standards of care evolved to fit the evidence that complications were so rare that routine post-op appointments placed an unnecessary burden on patients—travel, time away from work and family, and lost wages.

38. Kierkegaard famously observed, "Anxiety is the dizziness of freedom" in his 1844 treatise *The Concept of Anxiety*. Gordon Marino, "The Danish Doctor of Dread," *The New York Times*, March 17, 2012. For more on the thoughts of Paul Tillich, see his book *The Courage to Be*.

39. Patient journal entry transcripts.

40. Patient journal entry transcripts.

41. We are once again indebted to Gillian Frank, PhD. His book *A Sacred Choice: Liberal Religion and the Struggle for Reproductive Freedom Before* Roe v. Wade has not yet been released as of the writing of *this* book but will be available from the University of North Carolina Press. More of Dr. Frank's work can be found at www.gillianfrank .com#public-scholarship/.

42. Glenna and I are both deeply indebted to a former staff member, Patricia O'Connor, who now teaches creative nonfiction writing in the English department of The School of Liberal Arts at Central New Mexico Community College. An essay she wrote on her years of work

at our Albuquerque clinic, "Private Ceremonies," was nominated for a Pushcart Prize and later adapted as a TED Talk (TEDxABQWomen). Patricia O'Connor, "My Private Ceremony," filmed December 2014 in Albuquerque, New Mexico, TEDx video, https://www.youtube.com /watch?v=tnG2HNJ0hRQ.

About the Authors

Curtis Boyd, MD, is nationally known for developing abortion procedures and standards of care. He is also recognized for his expertise in pain management and minimizing surgery risk. Furthermore, Dr. Boyd was involved in establishing the National Abortion Federation (NAF) and is a founding member of the federation's board of directors. NAF serves as a forum for abortion providers and others committed to providing quality abortion services so that they remain accessible to all women.

Glenna Halvorson-Boyd, PhD, RN, served on National Abortion Federation's board of directors and as NAF's president for two years (1984–1986). She is an accomplished counselor, trainer, and consultant with a national reputation for her training of professionals in this field. Dr. Halvorson-Boyd has a PhD in human and organizational development. Her previous publications include the book *Dancing in Limbo: Making Sense of Life after Cancer*.